Cheer
the
F***
Up

Cheer the F**K Up

How to Save Your Best Friend

JACK ROOKE

In memory of Laurie, Sicely and Olly

To my best mate, Lewis, for always being there.

To my brother, Dean, for turning anger and sadness into courage and bravery.

And to my mum, Josie, who, despite losing the love of her life, somehow kept our home as warm and loving as it ever was. Who got nuggets, chips and beans on the table every day at 5pm. Who'd watch A Place in the Sun *with me on the sofa, a fag in one hand and a Müller Light yoghurt in the other – just riding the waves of whatever life threw at us. She'll get a free copy of this book, but I know she'll still go and buy one from Waterstones in Watford, because the shop makes her feel posh, so I'll see you in there x*

EBURY
PRESS

1

Ebury Press, an imprint of Ebury Publishing
20 Vauxhall Bridge Road
London SW1V 2SA

Ebury Press is part of the Penguin Random House group of companies whose
addresses can be found at global.penguinrandomhouse.com

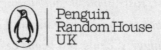

Penguin
Random House
UK

First published by Ebury Press in 2020
Paperback edition published by Ebury Press in 2022

www.penguin.co.uk

A CIP catalogue record for this book is available from the British Library

ISBN 9781529108248

Typeset in 9.9/15.66 pt Sabon LT Pro
by Integra Software Services Pvt. Ltd, Pondicherry

Printed and bound in Great Britain by Clays Ltd, Elcograf S.p.A.

The authorised representative in the EEA is Penguin Random House Ireland,
Morrison Chambers, 32 Nassau Street, Dublin D02 YH68

Penguin Random House is committed to a sustainable future
for our business, our readers and our planet. This book is made
from Forest Stewardship Council® certified paper.

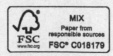

MIX
Paper from
responsible sources
FSC
www.fsc.org FSC® C018179

Contents

Contents

about this book

Hello you! Somehow you've ended up with a book entitled *Cheer The F**K Up* and who knows if that says more about you than it does about me! Either way, I am thrilled to be the hot young daddy of this new paperback edition.

You may know me from my live comedy-theatre shows, BBC Radio and telly shows on grief, or as the creator-narrator of Channel 4's sitcom series *Big Boys*. You may also know me as the guy creeping out of your flatmate Tom's bedroom at 8am and bidding you an awkward stranger's farewell on the stairs. (Spoiler alert – this author is a homosexual. SHOCK! HORROR! CRASH! WALLOP! God I wish he'd stop banging on about it already![1])

---

[1]   If you are a homophobe, please burn this book safely in an open green space away from low-hanging branches and children. If you're lucky, you might even see some cruising going on!

You may also not have a single fucking clue who I am, and for me, that is the most exciting demographic for you to be in.

I'm Jack and in 2019 I hid myself away from civilisation to write this publication, staying inside my flat with numerous tubes of each flavour of Pringles. I finally left my dark cave in March 2020 to hand in the final copy to Penguin and begin reintegrating myself into society. Then Ms. Rona had some other ideas and I immediately went back into the cave, this time with numerous bottles of Dettol spray to wipe down my Pringles. And whilst on lockdown, I realised a lot of the themes I'd written about – grief, loss and supporting loved ones in the toughest circumstances – became even more relevant.

This whole book is ultimately a comedic-memoir-meets-advice-guide, about losing my dad at fifteen, losing a close friend to suicide at twenty-one and losing a pair of Nike Air Max 95s on a Northern Line tube (Bank branch) at twenty-five. A real smorgasbord of trauma, I'm sure you'll agree. Many of the stories are taken from my Edinburgh live shows and explore topics such as, but not limited to: joining the 'dead dad club', confused sexuality, mental health, using sympathy to get free stuff, shagging, taking drugs, anxiety, finding the right counsellor/therapist, watching ITV daytime programming, surviving freshers' week, making shit songs on GarageBand, writing shit grief poems on Microsoft Word, comfort eating, parents, the Edinburgh Fringe, my deep love of Alison Hammond and the rapper M.I.A, property guardianships, suicide, masculinity, music festivals,

Contents

Grindr hook-ups, cancer, comedy, and most importantly – friendship.

This book is, above all, an ode to silly, loving, fizzy, stupid, unadulterated, messy, spontaneous, letting-someone-have-your-free-McDonalds-hamburger-that-you-got-with-your-NUS-student-card friendship.

I've rounded off a lot of the stories with advice guides full of tips from me, which all essentially boil down to 'how best to help a friend going through a shit time'. Some of these tips are designed to make you laugh and some of them to spark off ideas. I know that I've been that friend, had that friend and sadly lost that friend, and I think most of us have that one mate we're just that bit more worried about.

Brief examples of my friends who I worry about include:

- The one who divulges 'juicy' details of their sex life far too loudly in public eating areas.
- The one who has bought a few too many sequined clothes off ASOS in the hope of feeling footloose, when actually they just need some CBT.[2]
- The one who doesn't always order a chicken katsu curry in Wagamama.

However you may have that one friend – who could also be a relative, loved one, sibling or partner - where the issue is something a bit deeper and harder to broach. They may have lost a close loved one, may be struggling with their

---

[2] Cognitive Behavioural Therapy – more on this later.

sexuality, or might be feeling overwhelmed with symptoms of depression, anxiety and mental illness. I really hope there is something in this book that helps you feel more confident in giving them the best support whilst also looking after you. Quite frankly you could also be reading this book just to help yourself and if so, great! I've tried to write this so everyone and anyone is welcome, so long as you promise to start only ordering katsu curries in Wagamama, because it would be hard for me to trust anyone who'd order anything else. [3]

I can promise that unlike some mental health memoirs there will be no illustrations of dark rain clouds, clouds with sad illustrative faces in them, clouds with smiley faces in them nor any tiny sail boats on choppy seas. There will be no inspirational quotes, no stock image photography of people with their heads in their hands, nor any sentimental comment about how I hope this book can help just one person. That would be a lie. I hope this book helps at least 100 people and that one of them ends up becoming my husband, or else, really, what was the point? The only way I could reconcile with the self-indulgence of writing a memoir in my twenties, was to try and make it funny, silly and cynical at times, yet still sensitive, still a bit sad in places and hopefully still very useful.

Before I was doing any comedy or broadcasting, during my first year at university in 2012, I started volunteering at

---

[3]   This book is not sponsored by Wagamama, but I'm very happy for them to take me on as a brand ambassador if anyone knows anyone.

the suicide prevention charity CALM (Campaign Against Living Miserably). I've been a long-term ambassador, travelling with them up and down the country, from pitching 'free tea and talk tents' at festivals full of teenagers on MDMA comedowns to flying the CALM flag at their first LGBTQ+ Pride, to meeting Princes William and Harry in the gardens of Kensington Palace to kick off their Heads Together mental health initiative. I don't think either of those two were on an MDMA comedown at the time, but had they been, I would've had some reassuring words of comfort at the ready. (Mainly stay calm and focus your mind on something positive if you start to feel panicky, Harry.) I've also written columns for CALM, thrown numerous fundraising gigs for them, and over the years I've stood behind hundreds of pop-up tables giving out thousands of leaflets, badges and advice sheets, speaking to people who've been affected by various mental health issues and hearing about how they've come out the other side of it.

Though whilst I have some experience, I do want to state clearly that I am not a psychotherapist or psychiatrist. I'm just a boy, standing in front of a reader, via the medium of paper or audio-book, asking you to love him/at least read beyond page forty. (And then leave a nice Amazon review if you enjoyed it!) All I can do is share what I've learnt and trust you to take away whatever you want, so long as it's to help yourself or support a friend.

Ultimately, the reason I wanted to write this book is because I think we are living through a time period where the onus is increasingly being placed upon us as individuals to be mental health supports for one another. The clarion call of 'time to talk' has continuously increased in volume through mainstream conversations around mental health and yet Britain has increasingly long waiting lists for talking therapies, funding cuts to NHS mental health/ early intervention services and high suicide stats in some demographics – all made harder to tackle during the pandemic.[4]

Discussions that should be taking place in therapy rooms or within safe earshot of a trained mental health professional are now happening in our nation's living rooms and not all of us feel equipped for this or know how to help. With many young people unable to afford private therapy and treatment, I've heard more and more from loved ones feeling under immense pressure to 'save' those who haven't been able to access help when they've needed it. So whilst we've rightly encouraged people to open up, we haven't properly provided those hearing these admissions of depression, anxiety, mental illness etc., with the right reactions, solutions or things to say. Nor have we given people the strength to cope with any of their own anxiety, guilt and/or shame that may stem from someone else's sadness. And so there is a very real fear in being *that* loved one – a fear of getting it wrong, saying the wrong thing and making matters worse for someone.

This is why I've called the book *Cheer the Fuck Up*. Whilst that phrase can be an insensitive, lazy dismissal to

---

4   Recent stats from the Office for National Statistics (published September 2019) sadly show increases in suicide rates for young men, young women and those from more vulnerable backgrounds.

throw at someone struggling, I've also found it can be said out of sheer love, desperation, heartache, anger, exhaustion, despair, frustration and – most crucially – fear. We often forget how much love involves fear and the desire to protect those we love. And so in a schmaltzy, drunk uncle at Christmas wanting to give you good advice way – I really do hope this book helps reduce the fear.

Finally, I wanted these stories to be a celebratory tribute to my dad and my friend Olly and I hope that maybe it gives you some space to celebrate someone you've lost too. And who knows, maybe you will become that one reader out of a hundred who feels helped by this book and thus, as a result, will someday become my life partner. Good luck to all of us, I say.

Jack x

P.S If any potential husbands want to drop me a line, you can find me @jackrooke on twitter, or @jackdaverooke on Instagram.

growing up

As a child, my favourite book was the Argos catalogue. In the mid-nineties, me and my cousins used to have a catalogue each – the true bible for any three- to ten-year-old working-class child. As soon as the Autumn/Winter edition was available to pick up, we would all sit and scrawl circles around five or six presents with a biro, ranging from one big present (over £50) to a scattering of small presents. Then, our personal catalogues, which all had our names on, would be collected in mid-November, in time for the aunties to gather round a kitchen table like a coven, distributing product number catalogue codes to one another for purchase. This meant the Christmas presents could be bought in one place, in one efficient order, with everyone getting exactly what they'd asked for so that no one could 'fucking moan' on Jesus's birthday. It was total genius.

We would still make the holy pilgrimage to Watford's Harlequin shopping centre each Christmas, to traipse around staring at festive window displays before getting a

9

round of McDonald's Happy Meals in for the way home, clawing at my cousin Amy's eyeballs if she got a better free toy than me. But, as for our Christmas presents, they had already been bought, wrapped and name tagged before we'd opened the first window on our advent calendars, and with far more efficiency than anything I've been able to achieve nowadays as an adult man.

Around the age of three or four, you could have asked me about my family and I would have told you that I had two wonderful parents, Chris Evans and Vanessa Feltz. My extended family included glamorous Aunty Pat (Butcher), my northern Uncle Les (Battersby) and my various cousins Zippy, Dipsy and Wellard the German shepherd. This is what I earnestly told people on the bus in the mid-1990s, during a childhood spent obsessed with television.

In reality my parents were my dad, Laurie, a curly-haired black cab driver with a penchant for spearmint polos and Kronenbourg, and my mother, Josie, a fellow curly-haired multi-grafter who did any job she could get, with a penchant for starting the crossword in the TV guide but then asking if I could finish it off, because, even aged six, I was the better speller. (I should clarify at this point, as some of my friends have been confused by some of this: by 'black cab driver', I mean the driver of a London black cab, and not his race.) Together, these two curly-haired lovers from estates just north-west of London created the most curly-haired chubby white kid you've ever seen. I was like Roald Dahl's Matilda – a bit of a misfit. I loved reading and talking and irritating the fuck out of everyone with incessant lines of questioning.

I hated football and conflict and anyone not answering my every request for information. However, unlike Matilda, I was incredibly loved by my parents and only possessed one magical power – to spill drinks in public places with total ease, to the raging annoyance of my dad.

I'd say I had the loveliest childhood. I was quite lucky compared to my two brothers, who were born twenty-one and thirteen years before me, when my mum and dad were skint, grafting their arses off and in their teens/early twenties, still trying to figure the world out. I came about when they'd just turned forty, had some savings in the bank, a TV with all four channels and could spend quality time with me growing up.

As a very young child, I lived in a place called Mill End, a predominantly working-class area made up almost entirely of social housing and football pubs, with the junction 17 to 18 stretch of the M25 concreted bang through the middle. Mill End is next to little pockets of villages all harbouring million-pound estates, where famous people like Sacha Baron Cohen, Ronan Keating or Martin Kemp lived. One day my mum bumped trolleys with David Seaman in Tesco and had a hot flush. She had to sit down.

We lived in a block of flats next to a little parade of shops, a Methodist church where Fearne Cotton once attended a christening and a pub called the Happy Man, which burnt down on my eleventh birthday. Nowadays I think it quite ironic to name a pub the Happy Man when a lot of the blokes inside were miserable, overworked heavy-drinkers. Away from the pub, however, people in the community were genuinely very happy. There was more of a feeling of warmth in Mill End than many places I've lived as an adult.

It was in the kindness of smiles as you popped to the shops to buy some fags for a random aunty. In the silent agreement that the 'No Ball Games' sign was to be ignored at all times. It was in the opening of pub crisp packets at the side rather than the top so everyone could share.[1] It was in the scattering of kids' pedal bikes and mini-scooters around the park, where if you accidentally took some other lad's bike home you'd just drop it round their house the next day. There'd be no passive-aggressive jobsworth mum complaining about it on the local Facebook group, trying to suggest some six-year-old was a mastermind petty criminal. People just used their common sense.

My favourite thing about Mill End was that, every December, house-proud dads would spend far too much money on exterior Christmas lights in a neighbour-on-neighbour competition too 'tacky' for the middle classes and surprisingly quite camp for such burly tattooed blokes, all of whom spent hours erecting a giant inflatable bearded silver muscle bear in front of their gaff. (Otherwise known as Santa.)

It wasn't one of those areas where everyone had degrees or A-Levels or – as was the case in my family – more than three GCSEs, but emotional intelligence, resilience and a streetwise savviness was qualification enough. People looked

---

[1] I found it so strange when I got to university and was hanging out with middle-class kids in a pub that they'd buy a bag of crisps, open them and then keep them in their own hands, keeping the crisps to THEMSELVES! We before me please, this is not a Boots Meal Deal.

out for each other, kept an eye out for those who needed it and always defended those they loved, even if they'd maybe done something wrong, in which case you'd still stick up for them, but privately clout them round the ear for being a dickhead.

Sadly, Mill End was seen by some snobby types from neighbouring, more affluent towns as a bit of a shithole. A bit more rough. But like most places deemed shitholes, it was a *loved* shithole. It was OUR shithole. Most shitholes in this country are actually incredibly lovable places at their very core and I think parts of Mill End are a really brilliant place to live and bring up kids in a community setting. Other bits, like many places in Britain built up with council housing, have been sadly neglected by greedy councils and a lack of government spending.

However, with the status of shithole comes a sometimes silent or implicit suggestion by certain types that these places are devoid of culture. That working-class people aren't interested in literature or the arts. And this myth was best defied by one woman in my life: my Aunty Jenny.

Jenny was, and still is, an absolute fucking madwoman. She was the Hyacinth Bucket of Mill End, you could say – the main one in my family who regularly read literature in front of me and religiously listened to *Woman's Hour* on Radio 4, whilst also being a plasterer/decorator driving an estate car with ladders and power tools in the back. She constantly had – and still has – white Dulux paint in her hair and she can down a half pint of pure whisky like it's going extinct. She's a bad bitch, that's what I'm saying.

When I was a kid, Jenny used to buy me children's books, take me to see pantomimes or films or amateur theatre shows, and then we'd debate and critique the content of these in her Ford estate on the drive home. The only condition I had was that we listened to S Club 7 on the way there. She was adamant that class should not ever stop someone from achieving whatever they fucking well want to.

When I look across my family, all the women have had traditionally masculine job types, from my Aunty Marion, who headed up a bus depot in Bournemouth, to my Aunty Rose, who's a paramilitary sniper working in volatile areas of conflict around the world.

Nah, I'm joking. She's a dinner lady at my old school, but it's a tiring job that she's still doing at seventy years old, though the canteen can often feel like a volatile war zone if a Year 8 has lost their lunch card.

My mum, on the other hand, has had numerous jobs all throughout my childhood, from café worker to shampooing people's hair in a salon to office cleaner to barmaid. I have memories of some quite well-off kids asking me at school 'What does your mum do?' and watching their shock as I explained she didn't have one career – she was just a grafter. So many working-class women take on numerous jobs of varied skill levels because that's what making ends meet demands and that's what Mum had done for years before I came along. It's not about a job title, it's just about having enough money to put food on the table for whoever is sat around it.

Now, me and my mum have always been incredibly close. She's like a cross between Gwen, from *Gavin & Stacey*, and

Pam ... from *Gavin & Stacey*. If you haven't seen *Gavin & Stacey*, this just means my mum's the sort of person who looks after everyone and jumps when the toaster pops unexpectedly. And whilst she's the woman who gave birth to me (via forceps, sorry Mum!), washed my pants for years (sorry Mum!) and wiped Colgate toothpaste from my cheeks before school (thanks Mum!), she is also one of my best mates. One of the funniest, kindest people, with a hilarious tendency to get incredibly confused with masterful ease. For example, for her birthday last year I took her for dinner in a trendy restaurant and I found her in the gents toilets because she thought that the door which said 'L' stood for 'Lads' and the door with the 'G' stood for 'Girls' (sorry Mum!).

I feel very lucky to have been brought up with all these very vibrant, strong, no-shit women around me. Ultimately, women who'd had tough, difficult upbringings, without money or many further-education prospects. All of them worked their arses off to start families and gain more than what they'd had where they came from. And, on another level, I feel lucky that those women have also kept up brilliantly loud, unadulterated and filthy senses of humour and who can always banter as much, and likely with more ingenuity, than the men.

Growing up, it was often the blokes I saw who could be far too volatile and sensitive. I would see men down pubs who tended to conform to a strict masculine stereotype: English tattoos, England shirts, flying England flags even in off-years of the World Cup, newspapers open on a pair of English tits, England flag cigarette lighters – and so on.

As a child, I had an underlying fear of being around overt, strict and defined masculinity, because it didn't feel like something I conformed to. However, I still spent most of the late nineties and early 2000s trying to align myself with this out of a fear of appearing 'girly'. From ages three to eleven I'd be dressed head-to-toe in bootleg sportswear from Bovingdon Market, an abandoned airfield just outside Hemel Hempstead where you could get knock-off anything. I lived off pirate DVDs, bootleg Adidas tracksuits, fake Reebok trainers, Kelvin Klien pants and nylon Umbro shirts that would enhance my childhood puppy-fat breasts to the undeserving eye. I remember often thinking I was dressing like 'my hero', David Beckham, when in reality I looked much more like a dodgy Matt Lucas character from *Little Britain*, series one.[2]

I remember being so concerned through all of my childhood that I just wasn't boyish enough. I loved pop music, the Spice Girls, the various gradients and shades of the colour pink, and magic. My mum always tells strangers how I never wanted a dummy or a blanket as a child but instead requested a magic wand in hand at all times. I slept with numerous magic wands. If I lost a magic wand, my dad would go to the park, find a stick, wrap it in black tape and Tipp-Ex the ends and ... hey presto – Jack had a new magic wand. The gay signs were so obviously blaring out.

My brother Dean was the opposite. He's thirteen years older, so when he was eighteen and figuring himself

---

[2]   I should say that, in reality, my hero was Geri Halliwell.

out as a man, I was five, and I remember looking at him and seeing what it meant to go from boy to man. Often he told me that I needed to toughen up; casually telling me to be more of a 'boy'. He spent hours teaching me how to form fists, telling me throughout my childhood that, if I ever needed anyone or anything 'sorting out', he would always be there. All this when I was only six and the only trouble I ran into was the odd snidey playground comment about being too chubby to get to the top of the climbing frame. All I wanted to do was watch CITV's *The Worst Witch* with a mug of Options low-fat hot chocolate and sit doodling on a copy of my mum's *Take a Break* magazine.

Obviously, Dean never realised the impact these statements would have on me, but it definitely meant that I knew from very early on that I wasn't ever going to be your typical lad's lad, the kind of boy who gets called by his surname with a -y added.

I should say that, now, as adults, me and Dean have a much better relationship, despite still being *quite* different. I know he feels guilty about telling me to just stop being so wimpy all the time, but I also think his desire to toughen me up perhaps, weirdly, came out of love and fear, of knowing I was a bit different to the more 'laddier' boys and therefore might have it a bit harder.

And my earliest experiences of feeling different to other boys would always peak whenever we went down one place: the Mill End Community Centre for a 'family do'.

the family
do's

The Mill End Community Centre was an ex-primary school hall turned into a bar and function room, which hosted all the community's big events: engagements, weddings, landmark birthdays, Weight Watchers weekly weigh-ins, funerals and shit kids' parties. Think of the pub in *Shameless* but with fewer crisp options.

Every wedding, christening or even funeral of someone I barely knew would have a disco-lit dance floor. Most came with an old man stood behind it called Clive, who DJ'd for the night, interrupting each song with a banal anecdote about pop culture or sport or how this party can't go on all night, he's gotta get back to his wife![1]

Family members would always try to get me to play with all the other boys, who'd be outside running around the car park kicking a football, but, aged around five, I would

---

[1] Clive didn't have a wife.

always want to be on the dance floor, requesting Clive put on the Spice Girls – something that, at twenty-five, I still ask many DJs in clubs to do today.

These family functions were always soundtracked by sing-a-long party hits like Dexy Midnight Runners' 'Come On Eileen' or Barry Manilow's 'Oh Mandy' or The Police's 'Roooooooooxanne', meaning that the three women in our extended family called Eileen, Mandy and Roxy would get pointed, screamed and lurched at as soon as each song began. By the chorus they'd be violently dragged into the middle of the floor like a member of One Direction attempting to walk past a Topshop sale. Then everyone would shout the lyrics of the song at them and the women in question would have to pretend to be loving it.

And despite the non-consensual forced dancing, and my occasional terror of these events, there was sometimes a real joy in running around in a room full of extended family, even if I mostly had no clue how they were related to me. I loved watching everyone mucking about to disco-infused party music. The seventies and eighties hits of Michael Jackson, followed by more Michael Jackson, before an old fashioned shout-a-long song, like 'Is This the Way to Amarillo?', before swiftly returning back to the then king of pop. One of our cousins married a man called Mike Jackson, but no one ever dragged him kicking and screaming to dance and that's male privilege for you!

The other distinct sensory memory I have of Mill End family parties is the all-exciting finger buffet. There is nothing I love more in the world than a party finger-food buffet.

Once you get over the anxiety of knowing everyone *will* judge who goes up first, you can strut up to the buffet table and immerse yourself in the tapas of processed shite in front of you. I always recommend twelve-plus items as the bare minimum for buffet etiquette and *please* do not even think about returning to your party table unless you've brought back a communal plate of cocktail sausages.

My buffet highlights included: chicken goujons with a nondescript red or brown dipping sauce that was diabetically sweet, mini veg samosas too spicy for all the elderly white people, so there was always plenty left, a cube of cheap cheese on a stick accompanied with a pineapple chunk and, finally, some cut-up carrots or cucumber which you'd add to the far side of your plate to give the illusion of healthy eating. If you did begin feasting on any of the vegetables, some random bloke would probably call you gay.

As a side point, I would also love to pay tribute to the introduction of sweet chilli sauce as a regular character of buffets around 2005/2006, which changed finger party food for ever! Everyone wanted a dip ... except for my Uncle Saff, who was very suspicious of any food his palate was unused to. (One time he even refused to eat a lasagne I'd made, giving the reason that he didn't eat spicy or foreign food, which was ironic considering a lot of my family are half Italian.)

Now, the point I wanted to make by taking you to a Mill End Community Centre party was that there was one man in and amongst the more macho blokes who never made me feel like I wasn't enough of a boy. A man who didn't make me feel like I was a bit gay for eating a carrot stick. And even though he loved his cars and his pubs and no doubt probably enjoyed the tits in the newspapers, he was the one man who always seemed to accept me purely for me and didn't care what anyone thought.

My dad, Laurie.

school run

When I was around four, we moved from Mill End just up the road to a small town on the Metropolitan Line called Chorleywood. By this point, my parents were now both in their mid-to-late forties, had actually earnt some money and had managed to get a house cheap, right at the start of the mid-nineties property boom.

Now they had their own slice of the suburbs, with a back garden, a short driveway and some slightly snobby neighbours, who found the exhaust rattle of my dad's black cab to be far too noisy.

Chorleywood was a more affluent area, with the odd celebrity resident, many independent shops and a vanity twinning with a French town called Dardilly. Up until the age of eleven, I thought this meant they somehow found a town near Lyon which was completely identical!

I then went to a different primary school after nursery. Everyone else in my family had gone to a primary school right in the middle of the estates of Mill End, whereas I went to a village school at the top of a hill of very nice houses. I remember only being about five, but it feeling like a culture shock. There was one incident in my reception class when everyone was sat on the classroom floor doing story time and I came in late and asked Miss Lee for a pillow.

She replied, 'What do you mean, sorry?'

And I said, 'A pillow, please.'

She replied, 'Sorry Jack, I don't have a pillar. There's a pillar in the classroom but you can't sit by that, you must join the circle.'

In frustration, I shouted, 'No, I want a pillow!' pointing at what all my classmates were sitting on.

'Oh Jack, sorry, do you mean a pill-ow? A cushion?!'

I was pronouncing pillow like a cockney Victorian chimney sweeper. 'Pill-ah', like my dad shouting to Mum for an extra cushion whilst watching *Top Gear*. I didn't realise I dropped my Ts and contracted all my words until I went to this rather quaint village primary school, and soon felt like a 1939 evacuee from Bromley-by-Bow.

It was at this school that I made my longest-suffering best friend, Lewis. We met in September 1997, when Lewis witnessed me shit myself after I spilled three litres of poster paint on our classroom floor.[1] I started crying with embarrassment, falling to my knees on the reception classroom's low-pile blue carpet until the shitting came along

---

[1]   It was actually the exact day after Princess Diana died, but that didn't feel relevant to include in the main body of text. I was four years old and, to be honest with you, you could have put Diana, Princess of Wales, Jill Dando and Anthea Turner all in a row and, back then, I'd have never been able to say who was who.

as a secondary accompaniment to an already public melt-down. That was the first out of the three incidents, at the time of writing, where Lewis has sadly seen me shitting myself.

Despite this – and also at the time of writing this book – Lewis is still my best mate. We have been to the same nursery, primary school, secondary school, sixth-form college and university – and not even by design. We didn't actually realise until ten days before uni that we were actually going to be on the same campus. We've just always, always ended up together; whether that be in education or in the photo booth where we took the pictures for the front cover of this book. (Lewis got paid in a Wagamama pumpkin katsu curry for doing so – not a chicken katsu curry, because, bravely, Lewis came out to me in 2017 as a fully fledged vegan.)

My dad was the one who usually did the school run with me. He was a black cab driver in London, so he'd drop me off on his way to Heathrow airport, where he'd sit at the taxi rank for five hours with a Tupperware box full of warm cheese-and-pickle sandwiches – and not warm in a good way. We'd get out of the cab by my primary school at 8.30am, walk up to the school gates and he'd stand there with the school mums chatting shop and pretending to be one of the gals. The school mums loved him, much to my own mum's un-enthusiastic 'Well he's actually quite an annoying bastard to live with.'

I guess chatting at the school gates was almost like his warm-up routine, a way to acclimatise to a day ahead trapped in a black box of a vehicle, where he might have the loveliest conversations with total strangers from around the world for a transitory period of time, or he might end up driving a total cunt for three hours from Heathrow to a creative branding agency in Soho.

But at the school gates my dad was happy – happy to have a job where he could at least drop his kid off at a nice school.

On Fridays he'd pick me up at home time. All us kids would come steaming out of school and he'd be at the gates with all his school-mum chums. My dad was fascinating to my peers, because he was a cab driver and a lot of other kids' dads were bankers or solicitors or running to be a councillor. He'd make Lewis laugh by drawing a biro face on his index finger and thumb, cupping his hand and putting his false teeth in the middle, pretending his hand could talk, devising a new character for each toothy performance. I'm pretty sure one of the mums tried to book my dad as a party entertainer, but he swore far too much for that to be an appropriate booking.

I look back now and think how I was always really happy about my dad's ability to have lots of healthy, friendly relationships with as many women as men. He taught me the importance of having a mixed friendship group.

I remember another dad at my primary school once having a very loud dig at his son for hanging out with too many girls. The worried look on a father's face when he sees that his little boy wants to play mums and dads as opposed to 'fucking kick everything you see in the playground until it breaks or bleeds' is an upsetting phenomenon. It contributed to me also knowing that hanging around with too many girls either prompts the awkwardly polite 'Oh … he's just a bit sensitive' comment or the impolite 'He's a bit poofy, ain't he?' or, even worse, 'Ooh, he's a ladies man!' – all these comments describing a six-year-old *child* who can barely write their own name without getting one of the letters backwards.

As I'm writing this, I'm reminded of a beautiful thing that comedian John Bishop said on Jonathan Ross's TV show in 2018. Both men have been very openly proud and visibly non-fussed about having gay children, which I'm grateful for. John said: 'To the kids who are ten and eleven in the playground who are standing on their own who don't know where they belong or what group they belong in, and try to play up to something or feel isolated, and to their parents who think, "I don't know, my son doesn't want to play football, he doesn't fit in", I just wanna say, "It's OK." Just love them for who they are and allow them to feel safe, and then those little digs and the little knocks and the little abuse that they subtly get that we just don't know about, perhaps they won't penetrate as deep.'

It was a wonderful thing to say on primetime telly. And he was sat on a sofa next to four-fifths of the Spice Girls and HRH Kylie Minogue, so the gays were definitely watching. And whilst it did make me well up slightly and filled me with a feeling of love, it also made me think: John Bishop's a DILF. I would actually!

My dad shared this openness to parenting.

When I started secondary school, Dad would drop me off right in the school car park at the taxi rank, so people thought I was really rich and got cabs every day like the cool kids from west London. I'd royally wave, and call 'Goodbye Driver!' in an RP accent whilst he'd tell me to sod off and untuck my trousers from my socks.

I looked like a younger, chubbier version of him. Same unruly curly hair, same blue eyes, same crooked nose and teeth and the same overly expressive face when watching any film. Me and Dad watching a horror film were like Lee and Jenny who live in the static caravan on *Gogglebox* – all camp, terrified and shocked at even just a plate being put down on a table abruptly. I was a mini him and I spent the vast majority of my free time as a child out and about with Dad. Mum was very much someone I hung out with at home or at the shopping centre or at the big Tesco, whereas Dad was an adventurer – an explorer of sorts.

We would go on trips at least two or three times a month, visiting Dad's mates in different parts of the UK in whatever dodgy motor he was doing up that month to sell on eBay, or going off-roading around muddy tracks in a cheap red Ford F-150 truck he bought when I was nine.

Every Saturday morning from the ages of about eleven to thirteen, my dad took me in his cab to a leisure park in Watford with a bowling alley that smelled like children's feet, sweaty frankfurter sausages rolling on a rotating rack and employee malaise. I was a member of the Watford Youth Ten-pin Bowling Club and I was shit. I mean, really shit. There'd be seven-year-old girls bowling next to me getting five strikes in a row and I'd be throwing a tantrum about not having the barriers up. But we went every Saturday, always arriving 30 minutes late, having eaten a McDonald's breakfast just before so my fingers were so greasy from the hash brown I could barely keep a grip on the ball. Meanwhile, Dad would be hunched over, leaning on a wall somewhere, drinking a mixed-flavour Slush Puppie to try to cure his hangover from the night before, pretending he was proud of my shitty scores. It was love.

Eventually I got a bit better and was invited to participate in semi-pro youth bowling tournaments all around the UK, in the most exotic places, like Dunstable, Croydon and Hull. The other parents of young ten-pin bowlers tended to be over-competitive 'soccer mom' types, who were living vicariously through their children. I remember there was a dad called Mark Knobb* and I hated him. He was a jobsworth who believed you should clean your bowling ball with a small flannel for five minutes before throwing, and who gave people critical notes when they'd not asked for them.

One time he told me off for drinking a blackcurrant Fruit Shoot on the bowling lane and I just snapped and said the worst word for the first time. I was thirteen and, as the adrenaline pumped through my body, I thought I had whispered under my breath, 'You know what, Mark, you can be a real cunt sometimes.' Instead I'd angrily whispered everything *except* the word 'cunt'.

Everyone went deadly quiet and retreated to their bowling lanes. The blood pumped through Mark's body and shot straight up to a singular, throbbing vein in his forehead. I

29

looked at Dad, thinking, 'Shit, what have I done?' and he just went, 'Right, I think we're done with bowling for a few weeks.'

Instead we began to visit my nan and grandad in their flat in Harefield in north-west London. This is where my dad grew up, in a tiny two-bed upstairs council flat in the very corner house of an estate where, like Mill End, kids were always out playing, bikes lay strewn across grass verges, crisp packets clogged up pavement corners and flags of almost every nationality were tucked into bathroom windows.

Once inside the building, I would race up the stairs into their flat and immediately head for the biscuit cupboard. Here there were chocolate bars, Penguin bars, cereal bars – you name it, NAN HAD BARS!

Their living room was a shrine to the 1970s, with family photos everywhere – of me, my brothers, my uncles, my nieces and my cousins, with the biggest photo frame playing host to one of Princess Diana, for good measure.

My nan Sicely and I were incredibly close. She was a dinnerlady for about thirty years, and she had that kind and caring demeanour mixed with a 'no-shit-taken' attitude. Nan and I would just sit chatting or baking or playing Boggle or watching *Emmerdale* or weeding the garden for hours upon hours. We were so happy as a pair just doing our own thing. She was the woman who gave my dad his sense of humour and she would spoil me rotten with diabetic portions of fruit cake and Victoria sponge, along with a £5 pocket money allowance that felt like a £50k loan. She sweetly still carried on collecting Tesco Computers for Schools vouchers long after I had left school.

Nan rather vocally held a very strong belief that I was the one who had an opportunity to get educated – to pursue qualifications and live a life that she had perhaps wanted for herself if things had been different. She always took huge delight in how I was doing at school or in what I wanted to do as a job, like some sort of friendly, elderly UCAS advisor. She would later do something for me which gave me that dream career I wanted, without her even realising that she'd done it. I'll tell you about it eventually.

Me and Dad would often stop off at Nan's to say hey before going off to do our other favourite pastime which was to drive into London in his black cab and misuse his 'waiting to pick up elderly passenger sign' as a way to nab free parking so we could go for a walk around and explore. We made these trips so he could actually enjoy the city he normally only ever saw whilst sat miserably in traffic.

He was always very keen to show me the full range of the worlds that exist within the city that we lived in the very far top left corner of. He'd point out of the window at the multi-million-pound houses of Hampstead and Highgate, particularly the mansions on Bishopswood Avenue, owned by celebrities, footballers, Arab princes and mysterious Russian oligarchs. And then he'd also make sure to take me round the estates of Hounslow and Hillingdon; the high-rises where lots of his cabby mates lived.

He showed me 'the sticks and the bricks' in a concerted effort to ensure I knew how lucky I was – to show me how, geographically, there's not much of a gap between the richest and the poorest in our city. Later, I discovered that he also did this because he had a mate in East Acton who made really good hash brownies.

Being a black cab driver meant that certain theatre companies would send Dad free tickets to shows or exhibitions in the hope he'd plug them to customers via word of mouth. If the show was good, Dad genuinely would. Most of the shows were fucking terrible. I would love to say 'My dad took me to lots of live comedy as a child and that's why I am now a comedian', but it was quite the opposite. If anything, watching some drama graduates doing a low-budget comedy-musical about Tommy Cooper's on-stage death made me want to do anything but perform.

The one thing, that I was drawn to was music.

Dad often took me to pubs to see bands or open mics when I was a kid. Every journey in the cab was accompanied by his nine-CD changer, which held a mix of The Clash, Sex Pistols, The Jam, Lynyrd Skynyrd, The Eagles, Bruce Springsteen, The Who, Blondie, Van Morrison, etc. All the music that punctuated his early years became the soundtrack of mine.

By the time I was thirteen or so, I started to have my own favourite bands and our joint favourite were an act called The Holloways, known for a popular song in 2007 called 'Generator'. It went a little bit like: 'Dudda duh dah duh dah duh duh durgh durgh, do do do do do doo doo durgh' – and that's the only lyric I can write in this book without needing to get costly legal clearance from Sony Music Entertainment (SME).

Me and Dad went to see The Holloways four or five times in about a year, travelling to Oxford and Brighton, and twice in London. I was sneaking into 18+ gigs in pubs with Dad and having the best time, him letting me have a half of shandy every once in a while or a whole pint of Magners when we could get away with it. We started to go to Camden a lot, because it's home to a lot of London's music history and because my uncle was a caretaker at an office by Camden Market, where we'd 'illegally' park Dad's cab in the taxi rank and spend a whole day exploring record shops, flicking through vinyls, buying crap T-shirts with either *Mighty Boosh* characters on them or stupid touristy slogans, like 'Nobody Knows I'm a Lesbian.'[2] Our trips would also involve an obligatory dodgy £3 Chinese from a market stall called Bang Bang Chicken, where you were never quite sure what meat you were actually eating, but it was so deep fried that no one ever questioned it.

One time, aged thirteen, I wandered off down a Camden Market alleyway and, when I looked behind me, I realised this guy had followed me.

'Oi Curly, you good?' he said.

Nervously yet confidently, I replied, 'Yeah mate, I'm all good mate, how're you, mate, good, mate?'

'Yes, bruv, what are you after?'

---

[2]   Ironically worn by me, because nobody knew I kind of was one, bar a technicality.

This man then went on to explain all the readily available drugs he could sell me and the catalogue of other drugs he could order in at my request, should I give him my mobile phone number. Some of the words like weed and cocaine and ecstasy I understood, because of my brothers and because I'd watch *Footballers Wives* on ITV2.

Eventually I said, 'No thank you mate!' and skipped back down the alleyway to find Dad. I whispered to him, trying to be discreet.

'See that man over there, with the green leaf T-shirt? He just asked me if I wanted some of his spunk.'

Dad looked at me, smirked and said, 'I think you mean skunk, Jack, and please do not repeat this to Mum.'

On the way back from Camden, we'd stop at one of our local pubs for a swift one before home. There was The Sportsman, a pub on the Watford/Rickmansworth border, which was run by radical Irish lesbians, and which to adolescent me was just a place where everyone looked like a 2002 Mel C. They'd pour shots into half-pint glasses with no concept of measure or consequence, which, as an adult, I have found is the true charm of the Irish queers.

Then there was The Tree, aka 'God's Waiting Room' – a pub that always smelled like a hangover on a Sunday. It was full of men who looked like they were a bit lost in a multi-storey car park.

And then, finally, there was The Halfway House, where I remember one random man would prop up the bar and indulge himself with a spot of slagging off either students or gays or the missus or the immigrants or 'Tony fucking Blair'. We stopped going.

And then our black cab adventuring days came to an end, because Dad started to suffer from a back pain and the doctors discovered he had an abscess in his bum (really not a pleasant thing to be afflicted with). His GP said this was probably a result of years of being sat in his cab and so he gave up London to instead be a caretaker at the old people's home at the end of the road – something more local and less stressful whilst he got better. Then Dad had numerous appointments with doctors, specialists and nurses. He lost a bit of weight. And then some more weight. He complained about the pain again. He saw his GP again. He was getting really quite sick.

I don't remember all the details – partly as I was too young and wrapped up in my own world and because there was one big event on the horizon. For my fifteenth birthday present, Dad had decided we could go to Reading Festival 2008 together. At the time, this was my biggest dream. The line-up had Manic Street Preachers and Seasick Steve, who Dad loved, and Justice and Santigold for me. It felt like the moment my whole life had been leading up to – a proper festival, not just an open mic weekend down a shit pub.

Throughout my early teens I was convinced I'd grow up to become a radio DJ or have my own electronic band and get signed to a boutique Parisian-electro label or perhaps be asked to join the Klaxons. Dad got me a second-hand synth off eBay and I genuinely thought I would be the next

NME rising star if I just worked hard enough at playing the *Titanic* theme tune on a microKORG keyboard. It was very avant garde. The synth had a vocoder microphone on it and I spent hours pretending to be Imogen Heap, singing 'Hide and Seek' and repeating 'mmm whatcha saaaaay', much to my mum's annoyance.

Dad came home early from work on Monday, 31 March 2008, and we sat, ready and prepared with snacks, at Dad's big bulky Windows computer, refreshing the See Tickets page at 6.45pm to try to get elusive day tickets for the Saturday.

The rite of passage was: you went to Reading Festival for a day at fourteen/fifteen years old, then you went for the weekend with your mates at sixteen, and then, by nineteen, you got a girlfriend called Stacey and went to Kos instead, pretending you'd never even liked alternative music in the first place.

When we got the tickets, I was jumping up and down around the kitchen like I imagine Nigella's children do before Christmas lunch. I was beyond excited. We just had to wait until 23 August, which was 150 days away.

Just 150 days.

150 days

March–August 2008

When I look back, that spring and summer of 2008 was the last time I see myself as a child. I was fourteen. I was in Year 10 at school, devising plays in the drama hall, going into Watford with my friends to loiter and occasionally shoplift a Mexican chicken oval from Greggs. I was a teenage boy with no worries in the world, except one.

Mum was making me do Weight Watchers with her. Every Tuesday evening we'd sneak off for weekly meetings at a church hall in Rickmansworth, where a thin French lady would shout at us for spreading low fat butter on toast or for eating dried apricots ('zey ahre full of sugaaah, you imbecile') or for just generally having more than one chin.

Now, I've always been fat. I've yo-yo'd through the years, losing the odd stone every now and then. Being a big boy has historically been a limiting factor – I was never agile enough to get to the very top of the climbing frame at primary school, I was never attractive enough to get a girlfriend at secondary school to stave off allegations I was gay, and I was never quite slim-footed enough to fit into those Clarks children's trainers with flashy lights in the sole. Gutted.[1]

Weight Watchers and Slimming World have come in and out of my life like Kat and Alfie in *EastEnders*. On, off, on, off, in a spin-off set in rural Ireland, then on and off. What tends to happen is I attend the meetings, the weekly weigh-ins, lose two stone, feel amazing and three months later I walk past a Chinese all-you-can-eat buffet and the damage is done. I say damage – I'm not really obsessed with the idea of being slim or thin – I genuinely do believe you can be very fat and very happy. My issue is more that I can fall into really unhealthy traps with food and anxiety, and before you know it I've given birth to that additional chin and the mist of self-loathing descends.

Back in the summer of 2008, me and Mum were signed membership-card-holding Weight Watchers bad gals, with Weight Watchers branded ready meals, Weight Watchers peppermint chocolate cereal bars, Weight Watchers frozen sausages, Weight Watchers bread – even our scales had the Weight Watchers logo on them. It really felt like a bit of a cult, and one we were fully inducted into. Now, I don't want to fully slag off Weight Watchers here, mainly because every time I've gone to a meeting I always see people making new friends and feeling a sense of achievement. I don't want to be the person who scoffs at that, even if I disagree with elements of the model of weight-loss groups and find some of it quite exploitative. I

---

[1] They sell adult flashy trainers now on ASOS, but they don't go up to a size 13. Cunts.

totally get that they can be negative places for people, but the reality, for some, is that it sadly is the most physical experience of community they might feel in that one week.

Back then, for me and my mum, it became like a hobby. Losing two stone just as puberty was hitting me was a huge confidence boost. I started becoming more outgoing, wearing clothes that felt more like 'me' and even asking girls if they'd 'Wanna go to a Caffè Nero sometime?' (Then I'd go to a Caffè Nero with said girl and just talk about the female popstars we liked.)

I was also counting down the remaining days until my first Reading Festival, but Dad was still not well. He got some test results back and told me that he felt so poorly that he wasn't going to be able to take me and was going to ask my eldest brother, Alan, if he was available to. I shouted and screamed at him, throwing a tantrum at the possibility of not going. All I knew was he had an abscess, just a poxy infection, and it was ruining my summer before the last year of my GCSEs. I was livid.

At the end of the 150 days, Alan did indeed take me to Reading Festival. I don't even think I said goodbye to Dad the morning we left. I saw the bands I wanted to. I made friends with people in the crowd and added them on MySpace. I ignored my dad's call in the middle of the afternoon to see if I was having a good time. I also ignored his follow-up text. It hurts to write this because of what you've probably guessed is about to come.

In the following weeks after the festival, my mum was so stressed rushing about looking after Dad that she fell over and broke her leg. I then spent two weeks caring for both my parents, one who was just asleep all the time and pumped full of medication and the other who was in a full-leg cast. My aunties came and helped, but, when they went home, I was left with two people who were supposed to be *my* care-givers. As the weeks went on, it became clear that my dad was bedridden and was not about to get better any time soon.

One night in early September, I saw him shivering, tucked in bed with the heating on, under a duvet, but unable to stop violently shaking. I ran downstairs to tell my mum that it was frightening me, but we didn't have a clue what to do. We were all scared. And he got even more ill as each day passed. I would give so much now to be able to hug that frightened teenage kid who just wanted to fix things but felt so out of his depth.

I went back to school for my final GCSE year and everyone remarked how much weight I'd lost. How great I looked. But I didn't feel great, because everything at home seemed to be getting worse.

On 18 September, my cousin Amy and some friends took me out for some relief. We went to an in-store gig at Zavvi, the old Virgin Megastores shop in London, watched some bands and had a nice night. When we got off the train back home my aunty Rose picked us up, dropped me home, and hugged me just that bit longer than usual. I noticed everyone's cars were parked outside. My brothers, my other aunties. I walked into the house and went into the living room to find everyone sat there, in a semi-circle. In a way that you only ever see on *EastEnders* when some bad news is about to be given. They asked how the gig was and I said it was good.

Then my brother said that they needed to tell me something. And I remember Dad turned his head and couldn't look at me. My best friend in the whole wide world couldn't look at me. And I just knew. In that moment I knew what was coming. I felt all the hairs on my body rise to the ceiling. I felt all the adrenaline in my arms and legs and my chest started pounding. And all I said was: 'I don't want to know.'

I ran upstairs to my room. Slammed the door. My middle brother, Dean, who I'd never really got on with, came upstairs. He knocked on my door. I didn't answer. He walked in and sat next to me, putting his arm around me and telling me I had to come downstairs. And all I remember saying was – 'Is it the C-word?'

Dean nodded. It was kidney cancer. There was a tumour and it was big.

Me and Dean hugged for maybe the first time ever. After he went downstairs, I sat in my room and stared at a blank black TV screen – the news racing through my mind at 500mph.

And then I heard footsteps. The creak of the first step of our stairs – the sound where you always unequivocally knew who was *'coming up to Bedfordshire'*. It was the sound of someone as heavy-footed as me. I heard Dad come up the stairs and I quickly switched on my TV; a repeat of *The Vicar of Dibley* flickered in the background as he came into my room. He sat next to me. Put his arm around me. And I noticed he was holding a plate of buttered Soreen.

Now, anyone who's ever been on a Weight Watchers diet knows they push Soreen on you as essentially a way of getting some high fibre in your diet and some 'fruit' into your system. This is all well and good until you smother it in a thick one-centimetre coating of Lurpak, which is the only way to eat malt loaf. My dad hated Soreen because it got stuck in his false teeth plate, but I fucking loved the stuff. And so we sat, in silence, on the end of my bed, his arm around me, watching *The Vicar of Dibley* and eating buttered Soreen.

a statue

Every person I know who is the child of a parent who had cancer has a different story. A different interpretation of how that fear manifests itself and how it punctures your childhood bubble. Fractures your vision of the adolescence you thought you were going to have.

I very much feel my childhood can be split into three – before Dad's cancer, during Dad's cancer, and after Dad's cancer: the bereavement years. During Dad's cancer was such a short period of actual time, but it transformed me. It turned me from a boy into a man. From a child to an adult. Someone who had something vital cut short – the ramifications of which cannot be fully understood or easily articulated. To be the young child of a dying person.

Ten years later, I still feel those ramifications now. Sometimes I still feel fifteen. I'd love to call this book 'Fifteen Forever', but that is, objectively, an appallingly shit title. I couldn't do that to Penguin Random House. But it is how I feel almost every day.

Before Dad's cancer, the word 'cancer' was just that – a word. A word that carried the utmost fear, but that was obviously, clearly, categorically not going to happen within *my* family. It happened in soap operas or in sad Comic Relief films or in *Take a Break* magazine. Of course I was not going to be the child of a parent with cancer. Of course it wasn't going to happen to me, because I am me, in my life, of which I've lived fifteen years having so much control and I will probably have my dad until he is 103.

My dad will take me and my friend [insert name of female classmate I will ask to prom, hoping she pity-accepts to defer the outward reveal of my homosexuality] to the Year 11 school ball, driving us in the back of his trusty London black cab with a silk ribbon tied around the front of the bonnet to match whatever colour my date is wearing.

My dad will take me on my first official driving lesson at seventeen, outside of all the abandoned airfields and muddy tracks where he'd already secretly let me drive whatever banger of a vehicle he was in the midst of selling. Now he will be able to take me for my first on-road lesson and we will laugh at me being in the driver's seat and my complete lack of spatial awareness when it comes to parking. We will row over his impatience at how long it takes me to learn the simplest of manoeuvres and probably quarrel furiously over how loud I'll have Capital FM on. He will buy me furry dice as a joke to hang on the rear-view mirror of my first car, which he has always said should be a Volkswagen because the Germans actually understand the concept of legroom and it'll be the only car my pins can fit in.

A statue

At eighteen, my dad will take me for my first legal pint on my birthday, washing his hands of parental responsibilities and saying it's my time to look after him, the old git. He will watch me grow. He will see me achieve the life of an educated, successful person, reaping the rewards of all the opportunities he'd worked so hard for me to have.

And so you live your teenage years convinced of this, of your path, of the future and the rites of passage that come with each momentous milestone of puberty. And then, for me, all of a sudden, none of that happened.

No one even attempted to do any of those things with me because the trauma of what *did* happen was so huge, so consuming of any light or any hope, that I felt at times like my presence in a room became quite a painful emblem to everyone of the tragedy of my dad dying.

I felt like I became a statue. The function of statues is to remind people of the past, which was exactly what I did, because I still looked like me before Dad became ill. The boy who I was seemingly still existed because I dressed the same and sounded the same, but, in my mind, everything about me inside had totally changed. I had become someone stripped of all that innocence.

And somewhere in my head I see my own version of a statue. I see an image of a teenage Jack at Reading Festival 2008 with a cheeky Magners in a cardboard cup, who will suddenly come alive. And I watch this statue dancing around in a blue bomber jacket with muddy white Reebok Ex-o-Fit hi-tops, swaying without a care in the world. He's running from tent to tent, meeting total strangers in fields and screaming lyrics he has memorised at the top of his lungs. He's receiving free hugs off shirtless men who've clearly grown their own weed to sell. He is eating a giant hot dog with layers of mustard and ketchup, checking a festival lanyard clash-sheet to see the times of each band to ensure he can see as many acts as possible.

This is a statue of idealism. An image of me, not knowing that three weeks later he'd change beyond what he'd ever have imagined.

I feel obligated now, at twenty-five, to polish the statue of that kid. To keep him feeling loved and cherished, because that statue represents those happiest of days.

If you've lost someone too, and can empathise with what I mean about sometimes envisioning your past self before all the loss and pain, then, I know it sounds corny, but make sure you polish your statue sometime. Make sure you visit that person in your mind and remember what those feelings were like. Just every once in a while.

how to support a friend who's found out a parent or loved one has cancer

My general feeling is that, regardless of how old you are, finding out the news that someone you love is ill is incredibly painful. If you're under thirty I think it can be particularly difficult, because you may just feel overwhelmingly scared that you're not finished with that person/parent yet. That you still need them to guide you. To see you through. Here are just some tips from my own experience on how best to support someone who may have just had this really difficult news about a loved one.

1 Don't say it's all going to be OK, because, realistically, it might not be. It's very easy and feels quite natural when someone we love is going through something uncontrollably shit to try to reassure them that all will be fine. Sadly, cancer doesn't work like that. It will prove you wrong. Being the most supportive friend is often about just acknowledging how shit the situation is, trying to focus on any positives you can see, but mainly just being a huge comfort – someone who can listen, who can offer some sort of solace and escape.

2 Be open and understand that there might be some anger fired at you that isn't aimed at you. Be patient and empathetic to the varied levels of both fear and hopelessness that someone may be feeling after a loved one's diagnosis and know that, yeah, actually it might feel awkward at times trying to comfort that person, but life is awkward. In those moments they might need someone to listen to them, or just to sit in silence watching *Come Dine with Me* on a sofa somewhere.

3 Let them know you're there for them, but only if you actually are. That sounds a bit brutal, but what I mean is: don't overestimate the level of support you can give. Know what you can realistically offer as a friend, from the all-inclusive package of 'you can call me at 3am and I will answer', to the 'let me know and we can get fucked up in a Wetherspoons sometime'.

We all know that we have some mates who are more good-time gals – the 'Whatsapp at 10.30pm on a Friday night if there's anything fun going on' friend, or the 'ring at 11.30am the next morning to see if you fancy a dirty full English in the Morrisons café' kind of friend. Those people can be just as supportive and vital in their own way during a time of crisis, but just acknowledge what kind of friend you are. Don't say you're at the other end of a phone if you're not. Don't promise you'll do stuff that you know you can't.

4 Buy them something really fucking nice. Yes, it's superficial, but when the shit hits the fan, you want to feel spoiled in any way possible to make yourself feel that little bit better. Calmer, almost. Like you're still a normal person and not just a scared shell of your former self. It really can be anything from a petrol station bag of M&Ms to, I dunno, a cinema-sized share bag of M&Ms. I'm a strong advocate for M&Ms on demand in a crisis. But anything you feel fits, from a journal to a book,[1] just as a token of: yes, this news is shit, but I love you and I'm here and you deserve *temporarily* to milk this bad news in the pursuit of gifts.

5 Please don't go on about how your cat had cancer in 2012. Yeah, cats are cute and pets can obviously be very important in people's lives, but your cat's illness isn't relevant in the moment of this news. You'd be surprised at how many people will whip out their dead family tabby or Shih Tzu when you tell them one of your loved ones has cancer.

6 Don't pretend it's not happening. That's the worst thing a friend can do – to sweep away the momentousness of it all. Don't be a Pollyanna right now.

The overly positive 'gloss over the sad part' friends are often either dealing with difficult shit in their own lives or are perhaps struggling to support someone or they're just a bit cowardly and haven't been through anything majorly tough yet. We must forgive these people, because shit will hit the fan for them too one day. One day they will need us. A

---

[1] May I grossly take this opportunity to suggest this one. Thank you.

bit like how we all had to forgive those bloody Gryffindors for not believing Harry that Voldemort was back. Seamus Finnigan really needed a slap round the face in a couple of those films.

during Dad's cancer

18–28 September 2008

A little advance warning: this chapter is very sad. There are a few jokes peppered in here, some that came from my dad's mouth. But this is really about a tragedy unfolding. I understand if this may be too heavy to read for some and you might want to skip on a bit and come back to it. Please do read it if you can, though, because I think it might make some of you feel less lonely and help others be better informed of how to best support someone experiencing losing a loved one to illness.

As I said, every child of a parent with cancer has a different story. Some children are born with ill parents – they grow up in the shadow of diagnosis and treatment. Some children have years and years of watching their parent cope with cancer. Some children have months. Some children have weeks. I had ten days.

Me and Mum had ten days of knowing Dad had cancer.

Nowadays I flip back and forth in my mind about whether or not his late diagnosis was, in a way, a blessing in disguise. He wasn't suffering for long but, then again, ten days was never enough time to even begin to process what was happening. Not for him or for us or for anyone.

Those ten days feel very hazy in my mind. An amazing thing about our brains is how they can process a total life shit storm and zip certain traumas into a file pushed right to the very back of our minds. All I can really remember is the most heavy feeling of uncertainty and confusion. I remember going into my dad's bedroom the day after the diagnosis and everything feeling instantly different – like my dad had become as vulnerable as I was in the situation. This man of strength, my role model in life, had become so ill, so quickly. I remember staring at him, wondering whether or not I was about to lose him. Wondering what kind of battle we had on our hands.

You constantly ponder how much of a life sentence a cancer diagnosis is. Will he be cured? Will he have five years? I'll be twenty in five years and I'll still need him. What will Mum do? What will happen to our house? How will we survive? What will we do without him?

The questions come thick and fast, leaving you chaotically dizzy and, at the same time, violently numb. You realise that you really have no control of the situation.

The doctors had put my dad on a fully medicated course of pain management, mainly a brand of morphine called Oramorph, which does have its upsides, besides the pain relief. Dad's inhibitions went out the window and he started telling us exactly what he 'fucking thinks whenever I fucking think it'. His actual words.

Now, his doctors were at some fault, as they had caught Dad's cancer incredibly late, despite how he'd tried to alert them over numerous appointments that he was not well. His abscess had masked a much more serious problem – a tumour growing bigger and bigger on his kidneys. This will be the last time I mention his doctors, though, because it's such a sore subject and I don't want to resurrect the anger I had, but, in short, mistakes were made, as were apologies that just didn't feel good enough.

On that first morning after his diagnosis, I remember us going into the kitchen to make lunch. He asked me what food we had in and it was mainly just some mouldy cheese and tins of tuna. Mum hadn't been shopping due to her broken leg and the food my aunty had been dropping round mainly consisted of microwaveable curries and John West multipacks she'd bought in Iceland.

Dad quipped, 'Oh, I guess I'll have a tumour-fish sandwich, please.'

He started giggling.

'Congratumourlations on a fine decision,' I retorted, with a quick wit he was always impressed with.

I attempted to open a tuna tin and, as I'm notoriously cack-handed, with a double-jointed inability to properly operate any kitchen utensil, I went to give up on the can and pass it to Dad, but he refused to open it, demanding I learn. He pulled apart the can opener, showed me the inside workings and how I needed the sharp edge to click firmly on the can. He made me do it. I often think it was the last thing he properly taught me to do: how to open a tin of tuna. To this day I still struggle, but I won't just pass the can to someone else, even if it means I'm hammering a John West tin against a kitchen counter or, most often, just walking to the nearest Pret for a pole & line-caught tuna baguette.

The rest of that week of his diagnosis passed quickly. Hospital appointments all concluded that they needed to treat Dad quickly. He came home exhausted. Mum came home exhausted. I sat up in my room googling 'kidney cancer survival rates' and 'ways to cure cancer'. The kidney cancer survival rates were only good if caught early and the only thing I could deduce from my dad's condition was that it was not caught early. From my naive teenage Google search, the ways to cure cancer seemed to mainly involve sourcing cannabis, and Dad already had a steady supply of that from a bloke down the pub.

The final thing I googled was 'what to do if your dad dies?', which came up with nothing but relatively crap, clinical-looking childhood bereavement web pages, which hadn't been updated since about 1998.

During that first weekend, whilst Dad was asleep, me and Mum sat at the table downstairs in the kitchen in complete bewilderment. Both of us were just petrified and lost as to what our future was going to be. We held our heads in our hands, wondering what was going to happen to this man who was our entire world. I asked things like, 'So, is Dad going to die?' and she would say, 'I don't know, Jack. I just don't know.'

That Sunday evening my mum's best friends, Trace and Jackie, came round. I opened the front door to them and they wrapped their arms around me and I felt safe. Then I pointed upstairs to my mum, who I knew was up there, crying on the landing because she didn't want me to see her upset.

We were broken, under a claustrophobic amount of pressure. It had only been three days, but just having an outside presence come in and do the simplest of tasks, like Hoover the hallway or empty the tea bag bin, made things easier.

The next week I decided to try and go back to school because, in a way, it felt like a release – an escape from the tension, somewhere I could be a normal teenage boy for a moment. Mum kept reminding me it was Year 11, my GCSE year – the 'big one', upon which my future was seemingly decided – and that my brothers and aunties were around enough to help out. Whatever happened, she didn't want Dad's illness to spoil my education or the chance that I might be the first in the family with more than three GCSEs.

I went back into school on Tuesday, 23 September 2008. I told my form tutor about Dad's illness. He was very kind and informed my head of year. They reassured me that they'd support me in any way possible. And so I just got the fuck on with it.

For two days.

Wednesday, 24 September 2008

I woke up, got dressed in my uniform, popped into Dad's room to see how he was and he was sat up in bed watching TV. His eyes were a bright yellow hue, which I was told was just a side effect of the morphine dosage increase. I just thought, 'How does he look this goddamn awful and tired?' He was talking normally but about absolute bloody nonsense. He was telling me about some imaginary viaducts over our town and that if I didn't act now then the town was going to flood.

I said to Mum, 'What is he on about?' and she told me he was hallucinating. It was to be expected, considering the drugs circulating round his system.[1] Then he shouted, 'The fucking Romans are still building the viaducts and if they don't stop then Jack is going to be late for fucking school.' We laughed about it as she took me to school.

When I got home seven hours later, he had deteriorated even further into these hallucinations. I walked into his room and he immediately threw the TV remote square at Anne Robinson's face. He was sat up in bed watching *The Weakest Link*, calling her a 'nasty fucking cow and a mean bully'. And he said it in the calmest way. I found it hilarious until I told Mum and she burst into tears.

Essentially, his faculties were fast disappearing, like he'd gone mad or his real self was slowly drowning inside him. He was fading away amongst meds and what turned out to

---

[1] We didn't have viaducts in our town. I'd never even heard of viaducts until two years later, when there was a mega dramatic yet dreadfully CGI'd tram crash in a one-off live episode of *Coronation Street*. A carriage derailed from a viaduct and smashed through poor Dev's sweet shop! Gutting.

be the cancer spreading to his brain. But still, at this point, we did not know the severity of the situation.

Thursday, 25 September 2008

The next day a friend drove me to school and Mum and Dad drove to the hospital for a consultation. I remember we all left the house together, then got stuck in traffic, and Mum, Dad and Aunty Rose were in the car directly in front. Then suddenly one of their car doors opened and my dad got out and started walking along the road. My eyes popped out my head. My aunty jumped out and quickly ushered him back into the car. And that was when I knew he had fully gone. It had only been one week since diagnosis and it just felt like my dad wasn't inside there any more.

I got to school and I couldn't focus or pay attention to anything.

When I got back home, my nan and grandad were there instead of Mum and Dad. They'd been called upon to look after me for a couple hours as the hospital consultation was going on longer than expected. Nan put dinner on. Me and Grandad sat watching *Eggheads*. And then there was the phone call. My Aunty Rose was bringing my mum home, but not Dad. The doctors wanted him to remain in hospital. I watched my beautiful nan's face drop. She was being so strong, but she was as frightened as I was. The car pulled up and, as my nan opened the front door, Mum burst into tears.

'"He's got weeks," they said. He's only got weeks!'

The first person I grabbed was Nan, who looked like she was about to shatter into a million pieces. I held her so tight. Heard her scream for the first time. An eighty-year-old woman crying is one of the worst sounds you can ever hear. I held her so tight, fifteen-year-old me trying to tell her I was there, that I'd look after her, that it'd be OK. But I couldn't promise that.

Dad had been admitted that evening to a hospice. It was too late. He was going to die.

We drove to the hospice that evening and I sat on a mint-green leather sofa in a waiting room, picking holes in the upholstery – further widening work that had been previously started by someone else's anxious loved one. The hospice smelled like bleach and coffee machines that needed a filter change – a sort of stagnation. Everything there was geared for people being sat around waiting, because, I guess, waiting is exactly what hospices are for.

It was late so by the time the doctors were finished I only saw Dad when he was asleep. He had a bedroom overlooking a rather peaceful garden. I kissed his forehead and there was nothing for us to do, so we drove home.

Friday, 26 September 2008

I woke up. Overnight a huge commotion had started at the hospice. My dad had punched a security guard square in the face and tried to break out of the joint. Apparently he kept demanding to go home and he somehow escaped a locked hospital unit. At the time it was scary, but now I look back and think, 'Fuck yes Dad!'

According to the nurse, he had ripped out his drip and was found outside in the car park having used all his last strength to try to get back home to us. With two security guards required to calmly get him back to his room, his morphine dose was raised even further.

That morning, Aunty Rose drove us to the hospice whilst my Aunty Jenny was called to book the first flight back home from a holiday she was on. We arrived at the hospice and my Dad was in bed. He was no longer able to talk. I remember helping the nurses to give him a wash, roll him over, keep him cool. He could no longer take in fluids, so we had to administer water through a small blue sponge. I remember dabbing his lips, hoping he was taking in some sort of moisture. His lungs were croaking like the last few drops of a juice carton. The noise was horrible.

I decided to tackle it and help Dad feel more relaxed with music. That had always been mine and Dad's remedy and so I asked the matron on the hospice ward if it'd be OK for me to borrow her CD player.

'That's a lovely idea, darl. I've only Alison Moyet CDs, though, which probably isn't yours or your dad's cup of tea!'

She was right. Alison Moyet wasn't mine or my dad's cup of tea. Sorry, Alison!

I looked in my mum's car and found *The Eagles: Greatest Hits* CD. We played it from start to end, sat next to him whilst he lay there drifting in and out of consciousness, me hoping that these songs might bring him some sort of comfort. The nurse said he wouldn't be able to speak again, but he could hear us, and that we should speak to him. This was mad to me, because five days ago he was telling me how to make a tuna sandwich. We left that Friday night, went home and I dreaded what the weekend had in store.

Sunday, 28 September 2008

I sat with him, still dabbing his lips with these blue sponges. Talking away about how he was OK, that I was there and he was safe. We'd got so fed up of The Eagles over the past two days that I just started singing any song I could think of. I did an amazing *a capella* rendition of 'Sweet Home Alabama' by Lynyrd Skynyrd and he looked at me and smiled. There was a bit of him left in there. My mum came in and we'd just sit there, chatting away about nothing. Trying to make sure he knew we were with him. Anytime I'd then want to cry, I would leave his room, because I didn't want him to see me upset. I'd slide down the walls of the waiting room and just fall in a pile, sobbing, till a nurse or a relative came and picked me back up again. I just felt like the loneliest fifteen-year-old boy in the world.

Soon it was time for me to leave to meet Aunty Jenny, who had flown back to look after me. She was really who I needed whilst Mum was caring for Dad. And so I hugged Dad, who was mainly drifting in and out of consciousness, and just said, 'I love you, I love you so much.'

He had just about enough energy to lift his head upwards and kiss me on the lips. That was the last kiss I ever had from him. I'd decided that that was my goodbye. That was it for me. I was ready.

My Aunty Rose drove me home to wait for my Aunty Jenny. My mum, brother Alan and Uncle Clive all stayed at the hospice whilst I sat in our living room watching *The X Factor*. As soon as my Aunty Jenny's cab pulled up and she got out the car, I just ran out into the street and clung on to her so tight; it's the only time I've ever felt that I'd never be able to let go of someone.

Half an hour later, Mum returned home. Standing at the front door, she said, 'He's gone.'

I have to say that the first feeling I had was relief. A sense of calm washed all over me that the horror of the last ten days had ended. He wasn't ill any more. Dad drifted off to sleep at eight minutes past eight, with my mum right beside him, holding his hand, telling him to just let go. Telling him she loved him with all her heart. That she'd look after the boys. That he didn't need to fight any longer.

And, in a way, I'm happy, almost proud, that amongst all the tragedy and fear and sadness, his final moments were surrounded by nothing but love.

Josephine

That was quite an intense chapter and so I'd just like to remind you that there are some helplines and advice pages listed at the end of this book if you're at all upset.

I also wanted to remind you that this book is dedicated to my mum. This is because, whilst my dad continued to influence me throughout my adolescence, it was Josie who got us through it all. Who picked up both jobs, mother and father – all against the backdrop of her own pain.

After he'd passed, something immediately changed about mine and my mum's relationship. Something quite special. We shifted into a duo, with more binding us than just parent and child: it was like we became a team against the world. When she was broken, I would fix her. When I was broken, she would fix me. We stuck together like Phillip and Holly, even though deep down we were sad, like Eamonn and Ruth.

It's quite beautiful, for me as an adult man now, to look back at that time and remember how much I loved my mum and how I still adore her now. She is the ultimate symbol of resilience, strength and, quite frankly, brilliant comic timing.

So, off the back of that last very sad chapter, I just wanted to write a tiny page about Josie, so that you know that, yes, I lost Dad, but I still always had all the love I could have ever needed because I still had her.

how to support a friend who's just lost a parent/ close loved one

Tell them you love them.

Tell them you're there.

Tell them to drink water.

Remind them to be kind to themselves.

Remind them they are more than just feeling grief.

Remind them, in a *very* sensitive way, that they still have a future, even if for a while they can't or don't see it themselves.

Remind them that you're not too scared to talk about it.

Buy them biscuits. Not cheap ones.

M&S ones.

The ones that are round and covered in chocolate.

Or the Dutch shortbread that's dipped in chocolate, that would also work, but they're always on offer so ...

Just know that I know that those biscuits are *always* on offer so other bereaved folks will do too.

Keep them in your thoughts.

Keep them in your invites down the pub.

Keep them in the loop about the fun stuff in life that grief can strip away.

'Like' their inevitable Facebook / Instagram post / tweet about it all.

'Like' any angry rants about the world and remind them that they're not alone.

Give them your Netflix password (or Now TV, which is pretty good nowadays!).

Give them a hug when they need it.

Make them something silly – a collection of old photos, written memories or jokes.

Make them sit with you and sort out all their boring life admin, which they might need to catch up on without feeling alone.

Make them a lasagne.

lasagne

September–October 2008

Dad had been dead for five days and, I shit you not, we had seventeen lasagnes in the kitchen.

Seventeen lasagnes hand-made and hand-delivered to our house.

All of varied quality, taste and texture – seven-actual-teen lasagnes!

The oven dishes containing said lasagnes clogged up our kitchen counter space, stacked around like sandbags in a flood. All seven-fucking-teen of them!

I bloody hate lasagne now.

Our neighbours and a gaggle of school mums renowned in Chorleywood for being absolute home-proud super parents, the sort you'd see as a friendly contestant waving to camera on a trivia-based daytime TV gameshow, all decided that the way to show that they were thinking of us was to make lasagnes.

Sometimes they'd just ring the bell, leave their creation on the doorstep and run back to their car as if their lasagne were an unwanted child. A Disney orphan of a Loyd Grossman-sauce assisted pasta dish. I remember saying to Mum, 'If any of these have got mushrooms in, I'm gonna go fucking batshit!', which is weird because nowadays I absolutely love a cheeky shroom.

In total, me and Mum received twenty-six lasagnes, four shepherds' pies and a home-made sticky toffee pudding, so we started sort of tasting them all in a BBC Two-esque game show way, judging our neighbours' efforts before deciding a winner. Please remember this was five years before *Bake Off* took off. It was like *Bake Off* . . . for lasagnes.

Me and Mum would rank the lasagnes from one to ten on a chart we kept on the fridge, displayed with pride and held up by Ibiza and Torquay souvenir magnets. We would analyse each dish, making critical comments regarding the amount of béchamel sauce, the quality of the mince, the neatness of the layering and the texture of the pasta. Marks were lost if too much oil seeped out the base of one lasagne, or if there was perhaps a noticeable lack of grated cheese on the top. There is no excuse for stingy amounts of cheese – this is a lasagne, lads, not a portion of cheesy chips ordered at 3am from a shit kebab house in Nottingham. Always err on the side of *too* much cheese.

After the marks were counted, checked and verified on Mum's Nokia 6300 calculator, the winner was announced (internally) as Tracy Brooks from Park Way. We informed her of this accolade and she subsequently, religiously, began popping round with lasagnes, apple cakes and pretty much anything she'd ever whip together. This lasted for the next few years. I still sometimes go home to my mum's to a surprise slice of banana bread or a chocolate brownie, all from Tracy Brooks. God bless Tracy Brooks!

This leads me to the first and earliest accompaniment to our grief – comfort eating. Yes, my Weight Watchers summer flew straight out the window after Dad died and, in its place, came about six new biscuit tins, all happily doing a circulation around the house, dependent on who needed them. Dead Person + Tea = Grief.[2]

It wasn't just the kitchen which got taken over by bereavement. Our living room had flowers in vases on every available surface – if a vase was not available to host a fresh delivery, then a pint glass would be used. There were fucking flowers everywhere. Hand on heart, I can safely say there's nothing worse than your dad dying AND getting lily pollen on your favourite shirt. Nearly every single item of clothing that I owned had stains on them, so Mum quickly banned all deliveries of lilies.

The next weird manifestation of our grief was that I then stopped wearing my own clothes and immediately started to wear my dad's. I look back on this with such love for fifteen-year-old me, who was so desperate to capture and cling on to him. His clothes smelt like him – a sort of vintage denim musk mixed with a far too heavy dose of talcum

---

[2] Originally, my first Edinburgh Fringe show was going to be called 'Dad's Dead Put the Kettle On!', because we got through literally thousands of teabags in 2008 and also because I wanted sponsorship from PG Tips. I decided upon *Good Grief* because it took up less word count in the Edinburgh Fringe brochure.

powder. The feel of his clothes was like a tribute to him – everything very thick and constructed. I almost had to grieve his appearance, and to this day I still dress head to toe in denim most days, almost in tribute to his scruffiness.

As our extended family were doing the rounds of bereavement, the informing distant relatives, friends in other countries, fellow eBay community users who somehow all thought my dad was a legend, we all had to plan a funeral that we completely weren't prepared for. Me, Mum, my brothers Dean and Alan and my Uncle Clive sat around a table making a plan. It was too much for my nan and grandad to endure. They didn't deserve to bury their child, let alone try to organise it.

Dad had said to his mate Mike that he wanted to go to his funeral in a coffin on the back of a pick-up truck, which Mike was willing to facilitate, but my nan felt it was too much and was paranoid the coffin could slide out the back. So we agreed against this.

Then a lovely woman called Sue sent by the funeral directors came round to our house and declared herself a humanist celebrant. This is someone who compiles then delivers very individual-led funeral services that can include as much or as little religious sentiment as desired. Considering my dad wasn't remotely the 'Church of England' Christian his death certificate said he was, we opted for her to do the least religious service possible. Everyone attending was to come in double or triple denim. There would be rock music, poetry, funny stories. We only chose one hymn – 'All Things Bright and Beautiful' – to keep Nan happy. The rest of it was a Fun-4-All, not-a-funeral, because, despite all the trauma of losing him, the word that everyone continually used to describe him was 'fun'. He was such a joyful, spontaneous, silly presence in a room that the celebration of his life needed to be that too. That, and also it was what Nanna had in *The Royle Family* when she died.[3]

When I think about Sue the humanist celebrant, she was an absolute gift. She was from my dad's town, she rode motorbikes – actual bloody big fuck-off exhaust-type, powerful-engined motorbikes. (I think you can categorically tell that I know NOTHING about motorbikes.) She had this warm yet rebellious nature and wore leather jackets, but not like River Island trendy leather biker jackets that girls called Sarah wear to an office temp job, more like thick, waxy, punk leather. The sort you'd get in a back-street stall down Camden Market. She just seemed like the perfect person to pay tribute to the fifty-five years my dad had on the planet. Tribute to how fun he was. It wouldn't have surprised me if a steel grinder had fallen out her Jasper Conran handbag, if you catch my drift!

Sue sat in our living room about a week before the funeral and asked me to spew out all my memories of Dad. All the amazing things about him. All the stuff we'd do together. She recorded them all, took the best and funniest anecdotes to form a eulogy, and then gave us back everything we'd said as a family, written in a folder. And so we created a collection

---

[3] The 'Queen of Sheba' episode of *The Royle Family* is my favourite episode of television ever. Watch it!

of all our memories of him whilst they were fresh to us, something that, ten years later, I still cling on to. This is something I would definitely recommend doing for a friend who has lost someone incredibly dear.

Make a folder or a box, even just a drawer in a cabinet somewhere: something you can fill with all the things you want to celebrate about someone. Something precious that anyone can go to when they perhaps just need to remember.

Monday, 6 October 2008

The day of the funeral.

I woke up that morning in a weird daze, my head feeling very heavy on the pillow. I went downstairs and saw some of my family members in suits, ignoring the denim dress code, and I thought 'Fuck that'. I put on a blue bomber jacket, black Primark skinny jeans and my dirty white Reebok Ex-o-Fit hi-tops. I looked fucking great.

I remember the hearse pulling up outside our house and getting in the family 'limo' that I had presumed would be like a Year 11 prom stretch limo but was actually just a black car with some extra rows of seats. I had never been to a funeral before. I had no clue what the protocol was.

We drove for five miles to the crematorium, slowly following his coffin, passing all of the world that I'd grown up in. The pubs we'd watch bands in, the parks we'd sit in, the Texaco garage we'd shoplift pick'n'mix from. All my physical memories of him seemed to litter the roads of saying goodbye.

Lasagne

As soon as we were three quarters of a mile from the entrance of Breakspear Crematorium in west London, we noticed there were cars parked everywhere – vehicles strewn along the main road all the way up to the gated entrance. We saw people in double denim and band T-shirts walking towards the crem, hurrying their pace as they saw the hearse approach. And as we turned in through the gates, we were met with hundreds and hundreds of people – my dad's friends, our family, distant acquaintances he knew from pubs or garages, random men he'd sold a second-hand car part to – all of whom had come to say the same goodbye.

I remember looking out the car window and almost being excited for my dad. It was so overwhelmingly beautiful and touching. And in that moment I just couldn't be sad any more that day, because, after a death so unfair, this celebration of him was exactly what Laurie deserved. I felt so, so lucky that this man was my dad.

When I stepped out of the car, everyone looked at me, I felt a bit like Beyoncé when she's ... stepping out of a car. As we entered the chapel, Sue was standing there wearing double denim with a subtle grin on her face that said, 'Let's bloody do this!' It was like being at a film premiere or an awards ceremony or a product launch for a new Levi denim shirt collection. The vast majority of attendees couldn't even fit in the chapel, so they turned on the external tannoy speaker system and the whole car park and the road up to the crematorium heard the service crackling through. There were people just stood outside everywhere. It was like he was the Princess Di of Ruislip for one day.

Around 600–700 people came.

Throughout my childhood, my dad had said on countless occasions on car journeys, nipping to the shops listening to Radio 2 or when the 9-CD changer in his cab would arrive at one particular song that 'When I die, I want Lynyrd Skynyrd's "Freebird" as my funeral song. But not the radio edit – I want the full 17-minute, live from Steel Town, Pennsylvania, version to play, and I want everyone to sit through it all.'

So that's exactly what we did. I can still so vividly remember him bouncing up and down on the sofa listening to the 4-minute guitar solo in that song. I sat in that chapel smiling the whole way through.

We left and hundreds of people filed out; I had absolutely no clue who some of them were, but we'd all said goodbye in the one way he wanted us to.

We drove to the Harefield Football club afterwards for a buffet similar to the one I described earlier. Yes, there were chicken goujons. Yes, there was sweet chilli sauce. Yes, I was the first to get up to pile up a plate.

We went to his local pub after that and people sang and shared memories and passed round a cheeky spliff outside.

We drank, we danced, we hugged.

We loved each other. We loved him.

The next morning, the local newspaper's headline read that our town had been voted 'The Happiest Place to Live in Britain'. Me and Mum laughed and defrosted another oven dish of lasagne.

She said, 'Not round our fucking house, it ain't!'

And while she was right – things were terrible and the worst thing ever had happened – there were still these certain moments that flickered in and out of our initial grief when I felt this pure, unadulterated happiness – a gratitude to a man I only had for fifteen years, but who I could call my father forever.

bullshit things you shouldn't say to the severely bereaved on the day of a funeral

'Oh you must be absolutely devastated.'

'Gosh it must be awful for you.'

'You don't deserve this.'

'You were so close, weren't you?!'

'I wouldn't want to be cremated myself.'

'That's maybe the saddest funeral I've ever been to.'

It is amazing how British awkward politeness and our complete lack of emotional intelligence can manifest itself in the grounds/chapel/car park of a crematorium or graveyard. These are all things I can genuinely recall someone saying to me at funerals I've been to.

I personally think that, as a funeral attendee, you should go in with a funny or happy memory of the person lost. Or alternatively go in merely to support and help the person bereaved. That's what one should do at a funeral.

Don't dial up the tragedy or start mentioning other funerals. No one cares that this is the fourth one you've been to this year and it's only July. No one cares that the last time we were at this church was when Steve and Debbie got married.

This is a day for celebrating someone who was dear to at least one person at the funeral, so tits and teeth it (sympathetically, of course), and for heaven's sake don't park your Vauxhall Corsa in the way of the hearse.

back to normal

During the weeks of Dad's illness, passing and funeral, the world was also going through some hefty changes. It was the peak of the US financial crash, of the UK banks being bailed out by the taxpayer, the ramping up of the US 2008 presidential elections and the first year for Cheryl Cole on *The X Factor*. All this momentous history was being made, yet I didn't really know or care about any of it (apart from Cheryl, obviously).

The power of grief is such that it doesn't matter if the financial system of the most powerful country in the West is collapsing, if your life in your little bedroom just west of Watford feels like it's falling apart, too.

I had three years of school and sixth form left after Dad died. I went back two weeks after the funeral because all this was happening at the start of Year 11 and Mum kept protectively worrying that this would all fuck my life up if I didn't get back and knuckle down. I really wish someone who knew anything remotely about the employment world could have come along and said: 'Actually, mate, chill! This is GCSE Drama and English Language, it's not the be all and end all. Just scrape through to A-Levels and then smash them in the dick!' But no one said that. Please, please do say that to any fifteen-year-olds you know, just to depressurise the whole thing.

So, on Wednesday, 15 October 2008, my mum got my uniform washed and ironed, made me a bacon sandwich with the holy trinity (anchor butter, HP sauce AND Daddy's ketchup), did my tie up for me and then marched me off to try to become a normal fifteen-year-old again. I was absolutely petrified and relieved all in one.

I was, however, gutted that I couldn't now watch *Loose Women* every day at 12.30pm. Absolutely gutted.

magic
powers

I had quite an aggressive relationship with Santa Claus as a child. I truly believed he was the man who could make all my dreams come true. As a twenty-five-year-old homosexual, I've realised that such a thing does not exist. A *woman* will probably make my dreams come true, and her name will probably be Alison Hammond.

I became quite stringent with my parents as a kid that I needed proper time to craft my yearly letter to Santa Claus each December, a correspondence that would be presented in impeccable handwriting and left on our mantelpiece on Christmas Eve before I went upstairs to Bedfordshire.

In my early childhood letters to Claus, I would always ask for one thing: magical powers. I was obsessed with magic as a kid, as you'll remember from my obsessive need to have a makeshift magic wand on my person at all times.

Each year I would ask Santa to bestow upon me a different discipline of wizardry and witchcraft, such as: the ability to fly, the ability to cast spells, the ability to make Geri return to the Spice Girls, and then, the year after that, the ability to be invisible – a power I would later gain in adulthood just by being over sixteen stone in any London gay club.

Sadly, aged ten, my bubble was finally burst and I realised I was a fool for believing Santa Claus was anyone other than my drunken dad, who'd stay downstairs on Christmas Eve and, once I was asleep, eat the mince pie left out for Santa, take a bite out of the carrot left for Rudolph and then drink the four cans of Kronenbourg me and Mum had also lined up along the mantlepiece. Come to think of it, it was weird we left Santa Claus a four-pack of Kronie tinnies each Christmas Eve, especially considering all the driving he'd theoretically be doing.

One of the first Christmases without Dad, I asked my mum, 'What did Dad do with all the letters I wrote to Santa year upon year?'

She replied, 'Oh yeah, he cherished those letters, kept them in his bedside drawer.'

And I was so taken aback with how sweet it was that I asked if I could perhaps find them to read.

At this point she felt compelled to hold my hand, rest another hand on my shoulder and say, 'Babe, I'm joking. He obviously binned them.'

get out of class card

October 2008–July 2009

A couple days after I returned to school, a senior teacher called Mrs Rigden called me into her office. I was mildly nervous, as I thought of her as the sort of teacher who'd quite often flip between exuding a Miss Honey from *Matilda* level of kindness and compassion to suddenly acting like a very passive-aggressive *Come Dine with Me* contestant, the sort who'd ask for second portions of the chocolate and hazelnut parfait you made, but then only give your night a 4/10. *That* was the kind of woman Mrs Rigden could be. And you know what? I really quite liked her. I loved the drama, to be fair.[1]

---

[1] Whenever she got really, really angry, she reminded me of Peter Marsh, the UK's worst-ever *Come Dine with Me* loser. If you don't know, Peter famously lost his week of *Come Dine with Me* to someone mildly less annoying named Jane. As the final dinner host of the week, he announced her as the winner to the group with

Rigden called me into her mint-green, box-shaped office and sweetly asked if I was doing OK and generally enquired about how things were at home. She wasn't the sort of woman you could reply, 'Yeah, they're shit' to, but she was the kind of woman you could say nothing in front of and that in itself would speak volumes. She took out a red cardboard folder, got some pamphlets and told me that the school had an official policy to 'best support and look after students who'd ... ' and then she paused for thought and politely said 'been through *big personal upheavals*.'

I think this was one of the first times I realised that grown ups will desperately avoid – often to the point of going right around the houses – saying the phrase 'your dad died'. It's perhaps why, as an adult, I've always made a point to say 'my dad died', because that is pretty much exactly what happened. Call a spade a spade. Call a dead dad a dead dad. There's nothing wrong with the word 'dead', however, in the English language we have created (and I've done my research), over 200 euphemisms for death, because historically and culturally we are total emotional wimps.

I can remember people saying things like, 'Your dad's in heaven now', and I'd be like, 'No, he's dead.' Not unless he's

a vitriolic rage unseen on television before or since. He stood salty and stubborn, like a boiled gammon joint waiting to be carved, and began spewing out: 'Dear Lord! *Dear Lord*, Jane!! What a sad little life, Jane! You ruined my night – completely, so you could win this money, but I hope now you spend it on getting some lessons in grace and decorum, because you have all the grace of a reversing dump truck without any tyres on!!' It was absolute TV gold. You can watch it on YouTube. I watch it sometimes as an act of self-care.

sneakily taking refuge in a gay club in Charing Cross. My dad is dead. Please just acknowledge that he's gone.

Neighbours or sweet old ladies would comment, 'Your dad, he's looking down on you now', and I'd think, 'I fucking hope not, or else he's gonna know I had a wank over topless pictures of Eric Cantona on my Safari Private Browser.' My dad is dead. Let's just say that he's dead!

For me, the term 'big personal upheaval' is much more appropriate to whenever I've moved flats in London and found myself suddenly nearer an odiously sweaty Bakerloo Line train station when I used to be a mere 0.3 miles away from the sweet, tender loving care of the speedy Victoria Line. If you've never been to London, trust me – that's a big personal upheaval! A devastating one, to be honest.

Nonetheless, back at school I was quite relieved that she'd sat me down to tell me there was at least some sort of action plan to help take care of me in this weird bubble I was living in. Mrs Rigden then took me down to the Matron's office – a woman who mainly relieved a lot of middle-class children's anxieties with: 'Why don't you have a glass of water and then I think you should probably go back to class, Annabelle.' One time she caught me playing with a box of free tampons on her office windowsill and told me, in an almost cheeky innuendo-laden tone, that I'd 'soon realise why you should never play with a lady's tampon reserves, haha!' (To this day, I still don't know what the fuck she meant. Can any gals reading maybe tweet me an explanation of the joke, if there is one?)

Our matron was a kind woman – a calming presence in any time of panic and incredibly good at stabbing people with EpiPens who'd accidentally been near a Snickers bar. This was sufficient for me to believe she was probably qualified to help me and thus I trusted whatever action plan she and Mrs Rigden had in place for my emotional wellbeing.

They said that, if I ever felt sad or upset during a class, or if I ever felt like I just needed some time to myself, that I could flash a credit-card-sized piece of laminated yellow paper to any teacher, which would permit me to leave a lesson and go to either the library for quiet reflection, to Matron's office for emotional support or to call my mum to pick me up so I could go home (and watch *Loose Women*!).

This yellow card was handed to me, and I read in a rather disconcerting choice of IMPACT font that it said:

GET OUT OF CLASS CARD:
Please permit – insert name Jack Rooke here – to leave your lesson.
He/She may be feeling sad and in need of support.
They have express permission from senior management and
student wellbeing to leave lessons and report to Matron's office.
Signed – Mrs Rigden | Expires: July 2009

I thanked them, put the card in my Quiksilver wallet (the one every male teenager had in the mid-to-late noughties) and left. I was really pleased they had both been incredibly kind and clear that full support was available whenever I should need it.

As I was walking back to class, my internal monologue all of a sudden had a lightbulb moment, which went something like: 'OH MY GOD JACK, YOU NOW HAVE MAGICAL POWERS! YOU CAN JUST LEAVE A LESSON NOW WHENEVER YOU BLOODY WELL WANT! THIS IS THE MERE MUGGLE'S VERSION OF AN INVISIBILITY CLOAK. YOU CAN CREEP ABOUT WHEREVER AND WHENEVER TO DO WHATEVER THE FUCK YOU WANT WITH GRIEF AS AN EXCUSE! YOU'RE A WIZARD, ~~HARRY~~ JACKY!'

I showed all my friends the card immediately. Their eyes lit up with the same realisation of power. This card could go for one million Maoams stripes on the black market. It was the bereavement equivalent of a Nando's black card. And, soon enough, I claimed my free half-chicken – and by 'free half-chicken', I mean I misused the privileges given to safeguard my emotions via ... the art of truancy!

My first victim was Mr Adewolo, double maths – a cruel 90-minute session that took place on a Tuesday mid-morning, right before our lunch hour. Mr Adewolo was a lovely man, but he was relatively new to the school and English was his second language – I fear now that teenage me took advantage of this, but let's remember before judging me that *my dad had just died*.

In these maths lessons, I sat next to one of my best friends since primary school, Samuel Clifford – a boy I'd known since I was four, whose dad had also been good friends with mine. Sam was also a fellow closeted gay teen, who I'd rabble on to endlessly during class about the pop culture icons we loved, despised or pretended we thought were 'fit' in order to mask our homosexuality. Looking back, it was so obvious. We were *so* gay. Sam was gay in a drama prefect kind of way, and I was gay in the sort of, 'Well, Jack's not really straight, is he?' We didn't say we were gay to each other until six years after this class due to a whole load of internalised shame that I'll be delving into shortly.

In our maths classroom, Sam and I sat in the far corner on a table that accommodated just us two and our incredibly trendy pencil cases – which would change on an almost monthly basis, to keep up with the latest stationery fashions. Our little safe space was well away from the front-row Maths Lads – a group of sporty boys whose dads were all city bankers or stockbrokers and who clearly wanted their genetic and employment history to be replicated in their offspring, all of whom were either called Lucian (Luke) or Maximillian (Max). One time in maths, I can remember one of the Maths Lads making an off-hand remark, quite casually calling me a 'faggot', maybe as a schoolboy joke or maybe as a mean dig. I did nothing but just shoot him a disapproving glance and then quietly sit back at my desk, with the word swirling around my head.

Me and Sam, however, had positioned ourselves in this corner to be closer to the Maths Nerds – girls called Helen (Helen) and Marianne (Marianne), who we would persistently ask for answers from in exchange for being kind about their hair. (Even they probably knew we were gay!)

Sam and I were sometimes split up and stopped from sitting next to each other for infractions such as talking about the BRIT awards or drawing artful silhouettes of Amy Winehouse on each other's pencil cases. (Honestly, if we had been at school when Amy Winehouse died then we *definitely* would have taken three days of statutory leave for compassionate reasons.) But somehow, the next lesson, we'd always end up back together at our corner desk.

For my first implementation of my Get Out of Class card privilege, I waited until 25 minutes before the end of double maths to enact my powers. Sam and I were so excited that I was going to use the card. I stood up, lowered my bottom lip slightly, creased up my forehead and discreetly walked up to Mr Adewolo, who was sitting at his desk marking notebooks whilst the class were busy ~~completing a task~~ BBMing each other.

I said, 'Sir, I'm sorry, but I'd really like to just pop out for a bit if that's OK.' I showed him the card.

'Oh. Are you OK?' he asked, with genuine concern.

'Yeah, I'd just quite like some time out,' I replied, like butter wouldn't melt.

Mr Adewolo smiled kindly and nodded as I gathered my things and waved a fond farewell to Sam, who was grinning like a Cheshire cat.

I fled to the library.

I HAD DONE IT!

My dad had 'personally upheaved', and this meant that I now had, effectively, magic powers. But as I sat in the library pretending to read a Jacqueline Wilson book, staring at a digital clock ticking down until lunch, I realised I was bored shitless. All I had actually done was taken myself out of a class where I was rather enjoying spending time with Sam and gossiping about Lily Allen. I knew that next time I used the card, I needed to somehow bring Sam with me.

The following Tuesday – double maths just before lunch with Mr Adewolo again – we tried our luck. I took to the lesson a Lucozade Sport bottle filled about halfway with just tap water. Lucozade Sport comes with a weirdly designed sucking bottle-top, where if you squeeze the bottle hard it'll burst out a puff of air which in turn spurts out around 10ml of perfectly formed water droplets. These droplets, if squeezed in front of a face, can look to the untrained eye like sad boy human tears. It was a very scientific approach to deception and one that I am very proud of.

For this attempt at bunking, Sam was the one to actually go up to Mr Adewolo's desk with my Get Out of Class card, whilst I looked down at my notebook, acting visibly sad, with an overly wet face. In an Oscar-worthy performance, Sam negotiated a deal whereby he could accompany me to the library, as he was concerned that I was really upset. He said I needed to talk to a friend.

Again, a concerned Mr Adewolo, who didn't want to deal with any emotional breakdowns as he was already struggling just to cope with a classroom of teenagers, agreed to our swift departure.

We gathered our belongings as I kept up an incredibly convincing glum facial expression and then, as soon as we were out of maths, Sam and I raced down the corridor and continued running and running and running all the way to the school canteen, so we could be the first students in the queue to be served hot food. We did this a number of times thereon, each attempt involving us concocting a different excuse as to why I was having an emotional meltdown in class and needed to leave.

It was spectacular. It was deceptive. One could say it was a queer protest against the manufactured dictatorial concept of lesson times. (It wasn't, but ...)

This was, I suppose, the first time I had used my dad's death to get what I wanted out of something – a manipulation that would go on for years afterwards and become an award-winning Edinburgh Fringe show!

However, before any of you judge me harshly, there were genuine times when I did feel really sad in lessons. My usage of the card was mostly legitimate, as there were times where the pain and trauma of what was going on at home would catch up with me, or my schoolwork, or when just being in a room with twenty-nine other children who pretty much all still had living fathers just felt a bit much.

I remember in English class reading a story one day in which a character's parent died and I could feel the whole room start to look at me, to see what my reaction was. Perhaps it was my own paranoia, but I knew that there was a subconscious acknowledgement by my peers that I was going through something huge. I would immediately feel conscious about how I acted in a space where death – particularly the death of a parent – was brought up.

Lots of child and teen literature, film and storytelling features a popular protagonist character who loses a parent or parents early on in life. There's Harry Potter with ol' dead Lily and James (who I think actually come across as quite irritating in those mirror flashbacks in the films). There's Katniss in *The Hunger Games*, Simba in *The Lion King*, Ariel in *The Little Mermaid* – I mean, the list of main characters in Disney movies who have lost at least one parent is pretty long. It's a device used by writers to enable characters to relinquish the protections of a responsible caregiver, liberating them to go on huge adventures.

Meanwhile, I was stuck in a portable classroom just off Junction 18 of the M25. And for the duration of my time in secondary education, I used to go to the one place in the school which was pretty much discreet enough to cry it all out. This was the disabled toilet in the sixth-form block.

The reason I liked it was because it was more spacious than your average school bog. There was floor space to dump your backpack, a door-hook to hang up your coat. It was the only place you could take yourself at school where you could have proper privacy and not feel stuck in a tiny boys' loo cubicle with gaps above and below the door, hearing the fapping noise of a boy in Year 9 who'd just started to wank.

This disabled toilet felt oddly homely, and I would sit on the loo, lid down, and I'd burst out all these emotions. I felt so often like a lit firework, fizzing with all these feelings that would build up and struggle to escape until suddenly they'd hurl out of me and explode. (One time I did accidentally pull the red cord and I had to run away and escape mid-cry to avoid detection.) Once I'd finished crying, I'd usually go find Lewis or Sam, eat a pack of Maoams and just try to be a normal fifteen-year-old again.

My Get Out of Class card expired at the end of the school year, in July 2009. It's funny that there almost was an expiration date on my grief, but, come September 2009, I forged the card so it looked like it expired in 2010 to buy myself an extra year's worth of crying in the disabled loo. I was very resourceful.

Sam

In those moments at school where I felt really sad, Sam would always be able to cheer me up. One strategy he often employed involved us sitting around a computer in the library and him searching for 'This Morning YouTube blooper clips' (before YouTube got banned on our school servers).

At the time, *This Morning* was hosted by HRH Fern Britton and long-term silver fox Phillip Schofield, who'd both continually be cracking up on air and making euphemistic jokes about, for example, dunking beef. Then they'd go off to cook a linguine with a nude Gino D'Acampo, standing in a naked Greek god apron, making basic-level innuendos about spicy sausages and putting an Innocent juice bottle woolly hat on his bellend. These were the wonders of late-noughties daytime television.

I guess what Sam did, which so many wonderful friends can do, was to make me feel normal. Grief can so palpably infiltrate your identity, but Sam masterfully reminded me that, first and foremost, my identity was just being his dumb,

Celebrity Big Brother-loving, gossipy friend. I was his pop-culture aficionado. The person who would also bunk off school to watch *This Morning* with Fern and Phil if it had a great guest on it. Or just any feature with Alison Hammond (who was and still is our hero).

Sam and I would make up silly characters, based on school mums or teachers who we loved making fun of. We would do accents for days at a time, I think one week even speaking exclusively in an Australian twang reminiscent of Mr G and Ja'mie in *Summer Heights High*, going round school shouting 'Where have you been, bitch?!' and 'There's a paedophile in the school!' In a drama lesson once, we made up a character called Alison, who was fresh out of a Julia Davis sitcom – a dull, beige woman from Slough who was somehow involved in the 9/11 attacks and wouldn't stop going on about it. We were constantly creating alter egos.

We were these two non-laddy, non-sporty and non-combative British closeted gay teens. And those two boys are to be cherished. Those two boys are in every school in the land and they are protecting each other against sly digs from masc, sporty bullies and homophobic micro-aggressions.

Whenever Sam would catch me looking sad, he would quickly pretend I was a local celebrity around school – 'The Boy Whose Dad Died' – and that he was some fan of mine and he'd start showering me in fake compliments. And so I'd swan around these school corridors laughing, pretending I was famous.

Thanks, Sam.

GarageBand

November 2008

My mum and Aunty Jenny took me into London so I could visit the Apple shop. Mum wanted to buy me my own laptop with some money left over from Dad's funeral and, as a zeitgeisty gay in the making, naturally I craved a sleek white MacBook. The pinnacle of late-noughties cool.

For a reason I can't remember, fifteen-year-old me booked myself on to a free in-store seminar at the Apple shop on Regent Street about GarageBand – the digital music software that had become famous after Rihanna's 'Umbrella' went to number 1 for about 1,000 weeks in 2007, using a drum sample that came from a free GarageBand loop. Every music tech A-level student, wannabe dubstep producer and shit bedroom DJ started using GarageBand, as it enabled anyone to make relatively naff songs for free, despite having little knowledge of music or any talent at all. This pretty much described me.

I sat for 90 minutes listening to a man called Xander in the iconic blue Apple Genius T-shirt drone on and on about sound loops and drum patterns when all I really wanted to know was how I could make my voice sound auto-tuned like Imogen Heap on 'Hide and Seek', aka the 'MmmMmmM Whatcha Say' song.

On this trip into town, we also planned to see the Christmas lights of Oxford, Regent and Bond Streets. But, mainly, this trip would be the first time me and Mum had been into London without my dad. A city that had my father's life, career and identity sprawled all over it. Where we had always rung him to meet up in his cab or for him to drive us home. Facing the fact this was now an impossibility felt quite cruel, but we knew we needed to confront it eventually.

I remember us stepping out of the Apple Store after the seminar and hearing the distinctive rattle of a black cab taxi exhaust – an evocative sound when you've heard it every day of your childhood, both dropping you off at school and then pulling up outside your house each night as you went to sleep. It was a noise that sort of signified safety, that Dad was home – and then, all of a sudden, that sound stopped. It just vanished. Every time I walked around London for years after I would essentially hear him, any time a black cab pulled up anywhere close to me.

So, on this Apple Store trip, the three of us did the bravest thing we could – we hailed and got in a black cab, back to Marylebone station to get the train home. My Aunty Jenny sat on the flap-down seat speaking to the chirpy driver whilst me and Mum sat in the back holding hands, staring out at the city that Dad had shown us. When we arrived at Marylebone after a 15-minute trip, the cabbie wouldn't accept our fare.

We'd done it. Just one out of a million things ticked off a list full of stuff we'd now have to do without him.

The next day, I got my trendy white MacBook for £600 in the sale at the electrical appliance store Comet (RIP) on Watford's industrial park. I got back home and immediately got on GarageBand, piecing together some pretty shit songs with some pretty shit lyrics I'd written about loss. When I say 'pretty shit', what I actually mean is 'very shit'.

I wrote up these lyrics and bad metaphors into Pages, documenting the most challenging times of the initial stages of grief, sometimes into silly poems or stories or – worse – synth-driven pop songs. I hate to labour the point, but they were truly dreadful in a way that only 2008 electro-pop songs were (and still are).

I spent ages learning the piano on my keyboard – my laptop keyboard – trying to figure out chord progressions and what notes were where, all whilst fingering some equation of QWERTY UIOP. Then I'd watch endless YouTube tutorials about how to craft songs, building up layer upon layer of loops and sounds until I eventually figured out how to also make my voice sound something like Imogen Heap in 'Hide and Seek'.

I never went on GarageBand because I thought I'd one day become a music producer, I just knew I needed to focus on something that wasn't real life. Where I could compose and craft and concentrate on making stuff in a whole separate world. That was my catharsis, an outlet in those darkest hours.

And from a psychological point of view, it was also a sign of me retreating from the world. I put on a lot of weight again after Dad died, mainly through eating microwavable snacks in my room till gone 3am and sitting at my laptop, trying to artfully articulate how I was feeling by making songs in bed with a pair of shit Poundland headphones, thinking I was the James Blake of Watford.

But this isolation, this withdrawal from the world, whilst unhealthy in many ways, was also crucial for my understanding of the coping mechanisms that I'd need to get me through grief; the same coping mechanisms I still need to this day – to create and to write. Even if it's shit.

bereavement counsellor

Quite quickly during the bereavement process, I realised that, when I cry, it sounds a bit like Jimmy Carr's laugh. That arpeggiated, upward crescendo of a cackle that Jimmy Carr possesses is an incredibly unfortunate noise to create when you're weeping your heart out.

When my mum cries, she does this massive gasp before – like Pam in *Gavin & Stacey* – as if she's about to say something petty-dramatic, like: '[gasp] You'll *never* guess who I saw getting athlete's foot treatment in Boots.'

We'd often try to cry together, mainly on the sofa at night time with crusty snot forming around our nostrils and an episode of *Emmerdale* flickering in the background. One evening, after we'd had a really long crying session, where I had stopped crying but she had carried on, I turned to Mum and said, 'I remember when I was little, and I was sad about something, Dad told me that happiness can be found, even in the darkest of times, if one only remembers to turn on the light.'

Mum smiled and said through sniffles, 'No, babe, that was Dumbledore.'

Now, this constant on-and-off crying continued for weeks upon weeks, and at some point my mum realised we needed some coping strategies beyond our biscuit tin and the crossword in the TV guide. There was only so much that her leaning on me and me leaning on her could do before we'd eventually crumble. So for the rest of this chapter I thought I'd let her help tell the story of how we got a bereavement counsellor, who, in some ways, managed to help us.

Interview with Josie Rooke, July 2019

ME: Hi, Mum.

MUM: Oh, are you not gonna record me into a microphone?

ME: No, I'm just gonna record it with my phone 'cause then I'll type it up.

MUM: Oh, charming!

ME: No, Mum, no one is going to actually hear this audio. I'm writing a book, so I'll just dictate it in writing, like an interview in *Smash Hits* magazine.

MUM: Well, when you made that Radio 4 thing about EMA—

ME: (interrupting) It was M.I.A., the rapper. Not EMA (Educational Maintenance Allowance). That was the £30 a week I got in sixth form.

MUM: Yeah OK, M.I.A. When you did that documentary some woman came and properly recorded my voice into a microphone.

ME: YES, I KNOW! That's because it was an interview for the radio! This is a book.

MUM: Yeah, but you told me you were also doing it as an audio book—

ME: (interrupting) Oh, you're actually stressing me out! I need to get this done because I'm up against a deadline—

MUM: (interrupting) Well get on with it, then! You need the money.

ME: Right, OK, question one. Can you tell me again how it came about that we got bereavement counselling? I can't really remember. Was it through the hospice where Dad died?

MUM: No. Dad died and then I barely heard from 'em again. We tried to find some services, but annoyingly, because of your age, you fell in a gap, almost.

ME: Oh yes, I remember this vaguely. A lot of the child and adolescent bereavement support was either for young kids, aged 6–13, or young adults, 17 or 18 and older, and I somehow fell in the middle where there wasn't anything for mid-teens.

MUM: Yes. And so much of the support was also just online. It was just lots of videos and testimonials and I wanted to get you help from someone in person.

ME: I remember watching lots of quite sad YouTube videos of children in their living rooms being filmed talking about their experiences of grief. It would be like, 'Hi my name's Emily, I'm twelve and my daddy died.' And I would be like, well, Emily, at least you've got a Nintendo Wii in the background there.

MUM: Oh stop it, don't be so nasty!

ME: Haha, I'm not being nasty, it was just the reality of the situation. I remember watching some sort of support group for kids whose parent had had cancer for years and years and I just couldn't relate to any of them and it was weirdly frustrating for me. We only had ten days of knowing Dad had cancer. Back then I felt I had more in common with someone whose parent died in a car crash.

MUM: Yeah, it was a very non-conforming experience of losing someone to cancer.

ME: Do you mean non-conventional?

MUM: Yeah.

ME: Non-conforming makes me think we were rebelliously breaking all the rules of losing someone to cancer! Which I suppose, in a way, we were.

MUM: It just wasn't the normal story you hear. Normally, someone has cancer for a longer time and they know whether or not it's terminal. How we found out and that, all in all, only knowing for less than two weeks, it was just so tough. We couldn't begin to prepare for it. I think that's why we needed help, because all this happened in such a whirlwind.

ME: Yes. You did so well, really.

MUM: Well I had to. There was no alternative.

ME: So, how, in the end, did we get that counsellor? Through the GP?

MUM: Well, I booked an appointment and I told the GP that I was worried you needed some more support with all these emotions and that it was your GCSEs and all that. And she said she'd try and arrange some talking therapy for both of us but it might take weeks. And so we both left the GP feeling a bit deflated. Then a few weeks later a woman rang out of the blue. She was a bereavement counsellor called Gail, and she said she could do our sessions by actually coming round our house for an hour with us.

ME: Were you like, 'Whoa, Gail, that's a bit forward?'

MUM: No, I thought, 'That's handy, saves me petrol money.'

ME: And so when she came round, what was the process like?

MUM: Well, now this might sound mean, but I don't think she was particularly useful for me. She wasn't who I would have chosen to get support from had we had the money to. She was in her seventies, had kids and a husband, and whilst she had all the best intentions to help us, I didn't feel like she was right somehow.

ME: Yeah, I remember her sitting in the armchair whilst we were on the sofa and just the whole session feeling very awkward and static.

MUM: She asked me questions that I found difficult to answer honestly at that time.

ME: Like what?

MUM: Like, she asked, 'What did your husband like about you?'

ME: Right ...

MUM: And I couldn't say, 'My tits and me arse!'

ME: Haha, you should have done!

Bereavement counsellor

MUM: But just some of the questions she asked, I found that I had to be very reflective about myself, and that felt weird at that time. It felt too soon. I didn't find it useful.

ME: Yeah, I think she had a very soft approach and perhaps we wanted someone to just help us more concretely figure out some better coping mechanisms.

MUM: Also, you were in the room, so I couldn't speak to her about anything that I felt may have upset you. It was all a bit awkward.

ME: Yeah, that must have been hard. Having therapy as a pair is quite a different experience. On the whole, though, do you think she was useful?

MUM: No. (pause) Well, she was useful without knowing it.

ME: I want you to explain what happened, because I think she was ultimately very, very useful.

MUM: Well, she was quite a tall lady.

ME: I don't think everyone needs to know she was tall.

MUM: Well, you explain her then!

ME: No, I want you to! All I remember is she smelt like a mix of Strepsils and Deep Heat. She smelt very Vicks VapoRub, you know?

MUM: That's probably how I'll smell when I turn seventy.

ME: And so she sat down and the session began and we got chatting ...

MUM: Yeah, and it was all fine, but she kept wriggling in our armchair.

ME: Yeah, I remember noticing that and being, like, 'Hun, sit still, we're telling you shit.'

MUM: It was a wriggle of bloating, almost. Like she'd eaten a big baguette before she saw us. Like an Upper Crust in a train station.

ME: Haha well, from what I can remember, we just sat opposite her on our sofa, surrounded by a mountain of unwashed, tea-stained mugs, a stack of used scratchcards, an ashtray full of dog ends and a copy of the TV guide where I'd drawn moustaches on Sonia and Martin Fowler and given Peggy Mitchell bogies.

MUM: Oh no Jack, I would have definitely tidied up before she arrived. The TV guide might have been there because you always bloody defaced any front cover of a TV guide I bought. I'd get back from Tesco with *What's on Telly* and, before I'd even packed away all the shopping, you'd have already drawn a dick on Stacey Slater's forehead.

ME: That was my bereavement coping mechanism ...

MUM: Now look, I don't wanna speak bad of this counsellor woman, 'cause she might read this book.

ME: She won't.

MUM: But I just think she maybe didn't get us. We're not a sort of spiritual, chat-about-all-our-feelings type family. If someone's got a problem then, yeah, of course you gotta open up and that, but we're not an overly emotional family. She was almost very American and shrink-like for me.

ME: At one point she asked me to make a list of all the things that I found difficult and I basically just wrote down twenty-six people off the telly who I'd like to punch because they're too smug. Fiona-fucking-Bruce.

MUM: Oh I quite like Fiona Bruce nowadays. I think she's very good on *Question Time*.

ME: So come on, what happened when she asked to see a photo of Dad?

MUM: Well, she asked us if we kept photos of him around the house and I told her there were loads all by the mantlepiece. And so she smiled and she got up out the chair to walk towards it. (Starts chuckling) And she sort of hobbled over to that canvas picture of Dad smiling at Natalie's wedding. And she smiled as she was looking at it. And then all of a sudden ...

(Me and Mum are both chuckling)

MUM: She just farted. Didn't she? She just let out this absolutely awful loud fart.

ME: It came completely out of the blue.

MUM: I just remember thinking, I must *not* look at you, 'cause if I looked at you, then we'd both start pissing ourselves laughing and that would not be fair on her.

ME: I could see your shoulders bouncing up and down in the corner of my eye. We were both trying so hard to keep it together because of the seriousness of the session.

MUM: But it was just so, so loud and powerful. Like when you undo your jeans if you get back home after being down the curry house. It was a proper, you know, releasey fart, just as she was staring at Dad's photograph.

ME: At the time I believed in fate more than I perhaps do now, because believing in fate and signs can sometimes be the only thing that can get you through, you know? Helps you feel still connected to someone. And I remember thinking it was TOTALLY Dad who made her fart. It felt like a sign.

MUM: Oh, I still very much believe it was, babe.

ME: And then what happened?

MUM: Well, we'd had about 35 minutes of the session left and she got back in her seat. I can't remember if it stunk or not.

ME: It didn't stink, it just smelt like, you know, dust.

MUM: Haha! Stop it!

ME: She smelt musty, you know? I know she was very sweet and kind but—

MUM: (Interrupting) You are twenty-five years old Jack, grow up!

ME: And then do you remember how she said she had to leave?

MUM: Yes, I remember the session not being over and her sort of grabbing her stomach. And then she said we should wrap up early.

ME: Yes.

MUM: And then we both walked her to the door and she said she would email us about another session.

ME: Yes.

MUM: And then she left.

ME: Yes, and then what?

MUM: We just, as soon as the front door closed, we both just fell to the floor laughing. I don't think I've ever laughed that much. We were sliding down the walls. She clearly had, you know, the squits.

ME   I remember my belly and my cheeks just aching with laughter.

MUM   And then that was it. We never saw her again. But, you know, I do believe in a weird way, that if fate exists, Dad made that happen 'cause we needed so much to laugh. We needed it. And that's how we've always got through shit times. Even now. We're still laughing about it, eleven years on.

ME   Because it was such a loud fart!

MUM   Haha, grow up!

ME   You grow up!

Poor Gail the bereavement counsellor did actually email us after our first session to book in a follow-up. She apologised for her 'hasty exit', but Mum and I never took her up on the offer of additional sessions.

I guess the overall experience made me realise that both laughter and crying operate on the same spectrum. They are bedfellows. Physiologically linked. Have you ever sneezed and farted at the same time? I have and it was quite an affront! The same applies to laughing your head off and at the same time wanting to cry your heart out. Me and mum would often tread this line as our coping mechanism, trying to make jokes or quips to help us climb out of the sadness.

In 2017, I was on the tenth episode of Griefcast with the wonderful Cariad Lloyd, a podcast dedicated to comedic and honest conversations about loss. We had so much in common, having both lost dads at fifteen after a sudden cancer diagnosis. We spoke about how we both felt we fell into a gap in counselling services; how she was taken into a therapy room with tiny primary school chairs and dolls in it. How we both felt like the sudden deaths of our dads from cancer was almost like the classic magician's trick of pulling a tablecloth off a table, except the trick was cruel and everything just smashed to the floor one by one. Weirdly, speaking to Cariad was such an amazing gift. Nine years after my dad's death, it almost felt like therapy just having someone to talk to who has been through the same experiences, and could reflect on how all the nuances of a loss can affect you in different ways.

By the way, if you'd like to actually listen to the bereavement counsellor story, I recorded my mum telling it in my 2017 Radio 4 show, Jack Rooke's *Good Grief*, which is on BBC Sounds, should you feel so inclined to listen.

So yeah, thank you Gail.

how to help someone find bereavement counselling

A bit later in the book I'll be going into how to help someone get counselling/professional mental health support (talking therapies) in a more general sense. However, despite mine and Josie's farty experience, I would really really encourage anyone experiencing a loss to try to access bereavement counselling specifically.

Watching someone you care about going through a bereavement can be tough, because they may be feeling a fuck-ton of different emotions all at once. You may ask how they are, and one minute they're fine and joking around, then the next they've crumbled to pieces and have eaten three Rolo yoghurts in one sitting. The mind can so easily wander off and, as soon as you feel you're having a good week, you can wake up the next day and just feel much worse again. There are no rules, no consistent progress. These feelings can come in such strong waves, but any good bereavement counsellor should be able to help someone figure out how they can ride them out.

Sometimes, unfortunately, going through the stress of finding counselling by yourself can be quite tough. Thankfully, I've been very blessed to have had friends recommend services or routes to go down and so I will try to impart that wisdom for you and your loved one.

1 Firstly – book a doctor's appointment. A GP should be consulted if someone is struggling with a bereavement, because there are some free NHS services there to help – even though the waiting lists for them can be pretty long, dependent on postcode/local mental health trust. But it's important to see a GP first and foremost where any sort of psychological support is needed, whether it's regarding depression, anxiety, post-traumatic stress disorder or a bereavement. They can give advice and care when the trauma is causing physical symptoms of distress too. Some people develop anxious tics, migraines, night terrors or just lose or gain a lot of weight – you never know how an event like a bereavement can impact your physical health, so help your loved one actually book that GP appointment and check in with them that they actually go. Maybe sit in the waiting room with them. You can also go in with them, if they feel potentially unable to articulate their feelings without bursting into tears.

2 Secondly, this is the only time I'll ever say – get on Google! There are some brilliant counselling directories online, which host lots of different therapists and bereavement counsellors. The charity Cruse Bereavement Care has a brilliant website directory listing all the regions of the UK and their free-to-access local counselling services, with links. It's very easy to navigate and the website also has lots of information packs and testimonials about grief and counselling to try to reassure people about what they can expect from their services and to help normalise how someone may be feeling.

Cruse also have a free helpline on 0808 808 1677 (UK) and 0845 600 2227 (Scotland), which is staffed by trained bereavement volunteers, who can offer some immediate emotional support to anyone affected by any sort of bereavement who perhaps feels they are struggling to find help. Or they could just be having a moment where the grief has become overwhelming and they need someone to talk to. This helpline is open every weekday, so if you are worried about a friend, consider getting them to call in.

I get that sometimes helplines can make people feel embarrassed or silly, or perhaps they don't see themselves as the sort of person who needs to call one. But my mantra is: fuck it! What's the worst that can happen by calling a number? As long as it's not accidentally a sex line charging £18 per minute, then you'll be fine.

Also, with so many of these helplines, the person on the other end is often a kind volunteer who has their own experiences and journey, or you may end up speaking to a trained medical professional. Whoever it is wants to hear from those in need because, firstly, they volunteered, so they actively want to help and, secondly, they'll be bloody fucking bored if no one does call.

Jokes aside, I truly don't think anyone can ever go wrong by just plucking up the courage to ring up. They won't care even if someone starts crying straight away – they are super prepared for that.

3 If someone struggling has the finances to pay for private counselling, I'd suggest checking out the British Association for Counselling and Therapy's online directory. Costs vary depending on the therapist, but each counsellor will have their own website explaining how they work, what fees they charge and what to expect from their particular bereavement counselling sessions.

4 If you are looking out for a person who identifies as LGBTQ+, then there is also a brilliant online directory called Pink Therapy, which lists a wide range of private counsellors and therapists, some of which specialise in bereavement and grief for LGBTQ+ people. For example, the loss of a partner in a same-sex relationship or support if a transgender person has been affected by suicide, as sadly statistics show suicide attempts being disproportionately higher in the trans community.

Finally, as the friend or loved one of someone going through intense grief, sometimes it can feel so hard wanting to help someone in distress, but ultimately the thing that mainly helps is just time. I don't necessarily believe there is a strict chronological set of grief stages, but I do think we can all generally accept there are a few phases that people can feel at any time, without necessarily moving smoothly from stage to stage. All involve trying to process what has happened and recover from the pain of it.

How to help someone find bereavement counselling

As someone who's been bereaved and who has also helped friends who have suffered a loss, I think it's about trying to help someone:

- Accept the enormity of it. It's very hard to understand early on that the loss is actually real and you need as much love and support as possible to get your head around what has happened and feel like you can, one day, adapt to it.
- Understand that sometimes it's actually OK to feel overwhelmingly sorry for yourself or angry at the loss. For me, there's nothing worse than feeling self-sympathy. I have been there many a time and it can be really tough when you just wish that stuff hadn't happened to you, especially if someone's death was tragic or in traumatic circumstances. Sometimes you have to find ways to accept those difficult feelings.
- Help someone when they reach the stage where they begin to invest less of their emotional energy in grief and instead put more of their energy into something else. In other words, be there for them when they start to be able to move on with their life. Encourage them and remind them of their abilities and support them when the smallest thing can trigger those painful feelings of loss to return.

Any bereavement counsellor and any good friend should be there to help someone to freely and openly talk about, remember and *celebrate* someone who's died. This can sometimes be the only way in which you can then feel able and free to move on and progress with your life. Keeping it all hidden and locked away, not acknowledging it or talking about it, can often delay the grieving process and make it much harder.

It's also important to remember that not everyone who loses someone has had a good, close or positive relationship with that person and, in terms of the grieving process, that can be even more complex and hard to compute. In those cases I would really encourage someone to seek bereavement counselling, because it can be harder to know how a loss like that can affect your emotional stability in the long run.

In the same vein, it's also important to remember that someone can benefit from a bereavement counsellor at any time in their life/grief, even if the person they lost died a long time ago. This is why I don't believe there are chronological stages to grief, as such, because I have so often swung along the spectrum of loss. Even now, eleven years on, there are still days when I miss my dad so much. When I feel his loss so palpably that I have to stop myself from self-pitying and try to invest my energy into something positive, hoping to still make him proud.

Finally, I should say that, in terms of then getting a counselling session booked for someone – whether it's a support group or just one-to-one sessions with a trained psychotherapist – it's all about trial and error. Not every counsellor and their approach will be right for everyone. Essentially, be prepared for it to take a few attempts before you find a bereavement counsellor who is the right person to help provide those coping mechanisms and that non-judgmental private ear to listen. And try to encourage someone to have a few sessions before giving up. Not every bereavement counsellor is a farty one. Just mine.

bubbles

December 2008–January 2009

The first Christmas without Dad came like an unwanted text from a dwindling friend that you're trying to phase out. The feeling of: 'Urgh, Christ! What do they want from me?! No, I don't wanna catch-up. No, I don't think it has been too long. I was actually just about doing all right, thank you! Stop trying to get me!'

But then, instead of saying 'no' to this catch-up, you find yourself going along with it. It seems impossible to ignore the friend without being a complete dickhead, and it's impossible to deny Christmas is fast approaching without being a total Scrooge.

I'd read on numerous bereavement blogs how 'the first Christmas is really hard', and it was. It was exactly that. Three months had passed by so quickly, and now we found ourselves sat around the dining table with my dear nan and grandad, trying to make sure they could cope. Pulling crackers, telling jokes, trying to ensure they knew how much we all loved them, because I can't imagine what a Christmas is like when you have just lost a child, no matter what age you are.

My eldest brother, Alan, innocently moved into my Dad's seat at the Christmas dining table, a gesture so tiny in the grand scheme of things but one that represented such a heartbreaking transition.

The whole loss felt magnified during the festive period, what with all the constant messaging of family life, punctuated via advertising and seeing other people's Facebook photos of their festive family bliss. Honestly, thank God for the *Gavin & Stacey* Christmas special of 2008 and the videotape reveal that Stacey Slater and Max Branning had been having an affair on Albert Square. Without those two golden hours of Christmas television to distract us, who knows how we would have coped? At one point I was downing tubes of Cheeselets and Twiglets like a stressed mum necking red wine.

Dad would have usually been at home a little bit more over the Christmas period, which meant we noticed his absence even more. The house felt so much quieter without him. Some family friends from Portsmouth came up to visit us and brought with them a tiny Lhasa Apso dog. All of a sudden, me and Mum became obsessed with the idea of getting our own – someone who would greet us at the door, who could maybe give us some purpose and solace in the hard times.

The weeks after, we started to scour weird websites searching for second-hand dogs. It was a bit like AutoTrader for dogs. Or Hinge for dogs. All were listed with photos, personality types, hair colour – the usual dog dating stuff.

In the end, we heard of a family who were moving away from where our friends in Portsmouth lived and needed to find a home for a dog called Bubbles, Shih Tzu, blond. (Can dogs be blond?)

Bubbles was around five or six years old and all he wanted was just to have someone to stroke him, take him on walks, feed him and clean up his shit. Bit like me nowadays. It sounded delightful. We spoke to his owner – Donna, human, blonde – and we were all set for him to move in with us.

He arrived at our house by mid-January and we fell in love. He was chilled, rarely barked but would happily sit grinning on your lap, a bit like a dream Tinder date. We callled him 'Bobby', as he couldn't tell the difference between that and Bubbles and I didn't want to be shouting the name of some sort of weird children's entertainer across the park.

The week he arrived, we went straight to the big Pets at Home warehouse in Hemel Hempstead and bought a bed, toys and all the other accessories we needed. A few days later we went to Costco and bought a fuck-ton of dog food. That weekend we took him on walks and went to visit my dad's plaque in Chorleywood Garden Cemetery. I cuddled him, sat in front of Dad's plaque in the grass, speaking to my Dad about how I'd finally got over my fear of dogs, nine years after a German Shepherd rugby tackled me to the floor in a Harvester car park in 1998.

After a week of having him, Mum decided that we needed to get pet insurance, so we took Bubbles/Bobby to the local vets for a check-up. We paraded him up and down Chorleywood high street – aka the 'Happiest High Street in Britain', and people were looking at us – but for once not because we were the family whose dad died but because we had a new blond dog. And our new blond dog was adorable. And the vet checked our new blond dog over for a really long time before coming back to us and saying, 'I'm ever so sorry, but I highly suspect this dog has a massive tumour growing in his stomach.'

'What?' replied my mum.

Bubbles went in for X-rays and scans and a huge growth was found. Mum hadn't told me that for the whole week he'd been with us she had actually noticed spots of blood on the pillow he'd been sleeping on.

The vet suspected the new blond dog may have cancer. My instinctive thought was, 'The blond dog that we got because my dad got cancer and died has now also got cancer and could be dying.'

I went ballistic. I went ape-shit ballistic. I went Gemma Collins 'Can I speak to the manager' ballistic.

We'd had him for a grand total of six days and, in my rage, we forced the people from Portsmouth to come back and take away the dog and the posh new basket and the toys and the food.

I remember Mum saying, 'We could keep him, you know, he might get better, Jack.'

And I just stared at her and said, 'I don't want anything with cancer living in my fucking house.'

I ran upstairs to my room and made a melodramatic teenage angst song on GarageBand about how everything I touch gets cancer – a sort of heavy metal track with lots of scuzzy bass and guitar rhythms and crunchy loud drums. In the audio version of this book I will try and include an audio snippet here.

The day after Bubbles left, I went to Charlotte Brooks', the daughter of Tracy Brooks the lasagne winner, sixteenth-birthday house party. I went in an inflatable donkey costume and got horrendously pissed super fast, in the way that you can at fifteen years old, underage drinking in the comfort and familiarity of people you once went to nursery with.

In the kitchen, Sandra, one of the school mums, came up to me for a chat.

'Hello darling, how are you? How's your mum bearing up? I saw your lovely new dog on Facebook, I can't wait to meet him.'

And, in my drunken, tragic state, I shouted, 'Sandra, Dad's dead, Mum's shit and the dog got cancer. What do you think?!'

Me and the inflatable donkey were quickly swept out the room by my friend Lewis and on to the dance floor. My friends could tell I was devastated. I felt cursed. I felt like I couldn't escape death and all the baggage that came with it. I was given a glass of water, slumped on a sofa, and Lewis, Sam and everyone looked after me. Cheered me up. Sat with me till I was ready to go home.

We never got a dog again, but there was a happy ending. Luckily, Bubbles *did* survive, has reached a grand old age, and he is still with Donna today! But from our point of view:

Bubbles 'Bobby' the Dog

26 January 2009 – 1 February 2009

RIP (Rest in Portsmouth)

how to support a friend on their first night out after they've been through shit

A friend who may have been off the radar for a while and is finally getting back into the party/pub/clubbing world is going to need some support. Firstly, check they are definitely ready for a night out and not just feeling forced into one before they are ready. Anyone who has had time out from socialising is likely to feel a certain level of nervousness and anxiety, just at facing a room full of people, or may even potentially feel guilty for being out having fun. If you genuinely believe they are ready, here are some steps/tips on how to make sure they have a good night out.

1 I would ask if they want to come round yours before to get ready and/or to partake in – in the cringiest term in the millennial vernacular – 'pre-drinks'.

2 Get some decent quality booze in (not the cheap stuff that's tempting to buy in Lidl), then maybe light some IKEA tea candles or curate a fun Spotify playlist full of songs

from your late teens which you can both reminisce over. If you're my age (24–27), chuck in a La Roux track or a Panic! At The Disco sing-a-long for good measure. You're in the safe confines of your own house so no one but you can judge you. Ultimately, I'd recommend maybe buying some nice wine or chilled bottles of beer/cider (or some softs, if that's their persuasion), but if you start drinking something boozy, stick to that. Don't be whipping out the voddy at 10pm or arriving at a party or a club and switching to negronis. Be responsible – alcohol is a depressant and you've got to do little mumsy things to look out for your pal on their first night back on the town. You don't want them mixing bevvies and crying in the bogs of a club about their dead dad. It is *not* a good look.

3 Make sure you eat something beforehand. I know this is *super* mumsy territory, but trust me, there's nothing like re-introducing yourself to the world of frivolous nights out and then poisoning your whole system with shock amounts of booze and nothing to soak it up with. I say, be creative and, if you can cook, then make a cheap and cheerful pasta bake, or if not, Uber Eats some 20-piece share boxes of McDonald's chicken nuggets and then put them in really nice bowls. I love shit food in gorgeous crockery. Maybe decant some dips into empty Gü pudding ramekins, so it feels like you're really pulling out the stops!

4 Don't constantly check in with them if they're all right – just do it once or twice. You don't need to ask them every half hour or flash them a sympathetic smile/wink combo to check they're OK. I've been there with some very well-meaning pals and it sometimes just felt too much. Yes, someone may have been through a very fragile experience, but this is not a smear test – this is a fun night out!

(I actually don't know why I just wrote 'smear test' there. I've obviously never had one, but I can imagine they're quite delicate experiences and you'd often be verbally checked in on? Any vagina-owners who are reading this, please feel free to tweet me if this is not correct.[1])

5 Gently remind them at the start of the night that it's OK to go home anytime if they need to and then be prepared to go home with them. Have a cab or night bus plan at the ready should you feel like they need to get away. If you go for the latter, make sure you feel emotionally resilient enough to fight off anyone trying to steal your cracked rose gold iPhone 7 from your hands should you have both drifted off to sleep on the N29. If you can afford to do so, split a cab and get yourselves home and in front of food/an episode of *Broad City* as soon as possible. I think it's safe to recommend the sitcom *Broad City* as quite a good tip for positive mental

---

[1]   I once had my balls checked for a lump I'd found and my GP wasn't available, so I had to be assessed by the on-duty emergency doctor and it was SO painful, as he kept rigorously rolling my testes around between his fingers and thumb, persistently checking in on me throughout the assessment, which was kind of making it worse. However, this emergency GP then revealed that he used to be a military doctor in Iraq and Afghanistan and he would do this for all of the troops and, I'm not gonna lie, it was kind of a turn-on. Anyhoo – this was a massive tangent, get back to reading the list.

wellbeing, as it's a show about the importance of friendship (it's on Now TV!).

But, yes, remind your pal that this first night out is not about having a huge one, it's just about someone trying to find themselves again, being social and taking baby steps in doing so.

6 Finally, just remember that you can always change the vibe of a night out. Unless you've spent big, big bucks on something – which I strongly advise you don't at this stage – make sure you're able to alter your plans and do something different. Nothing is ever set in stone. You can always leave the pub at 9.30pm, or fuck off a club night and go to the cinema or go bowling, or just do something else that seems more suited to making a mate feel better. Maybe go home and YouTube search 'Vine Compilation' clips or 'The Best of Gemma Collins'. This is what I do when I've ducked out from a night out and I *never* regret it.

prom

Summer 2009

I went to my Year 11 prom with my friend Jasmine, one of the few Muslim girls at my school and the funniest girl in my year by a mile.

She was hilariously quick, effervescently so – always shouting some sort of gossip across a classroom or trying to teach me Islam for Dummies at break time. I started to notice that Jasmine always wore a headscarf anytime we had an exam, and in the queue lining up to enter our examination hall I once saw her sneak a tiny mp3 player up her sleeve, hiding the earphones under her scarf so she could listen to music if she got bored.

Her dad ran a local Indian takeaway, one that sold onion bhajis that tasted like heaven. Perfectly crisp, not stodgy or doused in colouring, they were perhaps the best thing about living in my town. After my dad died, Jasmine would bring me in the restaurant's leftover onion bhajis from the night before in a thermos bag, which I kept in my locker, sweating away, eventually stinking out the whole Year 11 corridor. It was another brilliant perk of being bereaved.

We decided quite early on in 2009 that we would go to prom together. We wanted our outfits to make a statement and to include wearing as much gold as possible – and we nailed it! I had a gold tie, some gold skinny pointed shoes I'd bought from a Chinese warehouse on eBay, and she wore a gorgeous red and gold sari with bangles and chains to match. We had to have our photo taken outside the school hall and I remember watching all the other prom couples before us. The more athletic boys all putting their hands on young female teenage waists. The parents with crossed arms on chests, sighing at perfect depictions of young love. Then there was me and Jasmine. For our prom photo, I was pretty sure we just wanted to flip the bird and make a silly face, but instead we conformed to that standard prom pose. Putting my hands on Jasmine's waist felt strange, forced almost. As we stood taking our photos, I remember touching her, and the uncomfortable thought creeping into my head: 'Yeah ... I'm gay.'

Would I have rather gone to prom with a boy? In theory, maybe, but really the only person I wanted to go with in my year was Jasmine. She represented, to me, a rebellious spirit, a very kind heart and a lifetime supply of bhajis.

A few months after prom came the day we collected our GCSE results. This, coincidentally, was the same morning that me and ten friends were taking the cultural pilgrimage of teenagers from inside and around the M25 – Reading Festival, 2009.

I was nervous about both. Firstly, I'd be collecting my first set of major exam results and, secondly because it had always been mine and dad's plan to go to that festival together. It felt bittersweet going without him.

I turned up to the exam hall already in my wellies, prepared for festival mud, opened the exam board letter and saw my results. They spelt B,B,B,A,A,A,A STAR,D – D in Spanish, A Star in English language!

My mum was overjoyed. I was overjoyed. It was better than my predictions and I had safely gotten into sixth form to do my A levels.

I celebrated in fields all weekend, listening to Florence and the Machine and doing covers of her songs by our campfire with a ukulele. It was very 2009. I think some of my friends who came along knew that Dad was supposed to have taken me the year before but was too ill, and so they all made sure I had the best time. That someone was always around to come and see the bands I wanted to see or to stay with me in my cheap £10 Asda pop-up tent, which we soon discovered was NOT WATERPROOF. I was very lucky to have them looking out for me.

I started sixth form the next month, and suddenly Dad's one-year anniversary crept up; silently, fast. I started to realise it was coming and felt all the fear and dread that came with it start filling up my shoulders. The end of September is such a shit time anyway, when the daylight starts to roll away and the temperature dips to give out those first batches of common colds.

Ten years later and it's hard to remember exactly how I felt at the time, as the first year without Dad came to a conclusion. I was a dedicated Facebook user, and I have scrolled back through my timeline to see what I'd posted on the date of his one-year anniversary. I thought maybe I had written some wise words about what I'd learnt in that year of loss, perhaps a heartfelt message to my dad to get some emotions off my chest. So often people post on Facebook in the hope that other people might relate to something (or just have a spare room in their flat), but I didn't know any other fifteen/sixteen-year-olds with dead parents at the time. There was just nothing on the same level. Divorces weren't the same, nor were dead pets.

I did, in the end, find a Facebook post from the day of the one-year anniversary of Dad's death, and it's one that makes my heart swell for how innocent sixteen-year-old me was on Facebook:

> 'Walking to drama lesson with Sam LOL. Postin dis on my new blackberry!!!!?!?!??!?! Go on & Add ma BBM pin 2131BA3A'
>
> 29 likes, 16 comments

Nothing apt at all, but, at the same time, exactly what I needed to be posting. Just being a normal teenager full of excitement at having their first BlackBerry in 2009. And I know that receiving more than four likes would have meant the world to sixteen-year-old me.

how to help a loved one on a painful anniversary

Anniversaries can be such a painful trigger for thoughts of how much a person is missed and the hole they may have created in someone's life. So, firstly, don't ignore the day when it comes around. You may want to take a sensitive approach and not make a song and dance about it, but whatever you do, make sure you use it as an opportunity to comfort someone. Send a brief text, a 'thinking of you'.

If you know the anniversary is coming up for someone, then I'd recommend finding out what they want to do on the actual day, if anything. Similar to the advice about helping someone have their first night out, remind them that their plans can always change depending on how they feel in the moment. Reassure them that they are in control of their emotions, because so often grief can make you feel like you're stripped of that power and autonomy.

They might want to do something quite conventional and respectable, like take flowers to a grave/plaque – in which case, do they want some company? Every year me and my mum leave some flowers and a bottle of Becks by Dad's plaque – even if a roaming teenage boozer drinks it, at least someone's having a good time.

Someone bereaved may also want to do something bigger, like go to a gig, visit some friends or have a slap-up chicken katsu curry (with extra sauce on the side) from Wagamama. (This will always be my personal choice of anniversary activity.) If there's a place, activity, favourite pub or location that has some significance in someone's relationship with the person they lost, perhaps you can help them create some sort of ritual, a yearly pilgrimage that can mark that anniversary. A place that reminds your friend of good times with whoever is gone.

They may want to go away, even – fuck it, anything that can take their mind off of it, if that's what they want (and if affordable). They might just feel like taking the chance to spend quality time with people who are still here. Who are still around to be loved.

I really enjoy looking at old photos and videos of my dad on these anniversaries. Most of all, on his anniversary I listen to his favourite music. Those songs I played in the hospice in his last moments. Songs that take me straight back to the back seat of his black cab.

If you are the bereaved person, I think it's important to treat oneself, not only with the indulgence of eating a chicken katsu but by properly celebrating your own resilience as each anniversary passes. It's good that you can see how far you've come without feeling guilty. Though also, on that day, it's totally fine to be anxious about how you may still have a way to go in that grieving process. In any case, getting as much support, in the form of great friends, family and others, is so important.

Anniversaries can be dreaded, but they don't have to be awful. They can be a comfort, a strength and a reminder of love.

sixth form

When I was a teenager, people would say to me: 'These are the happiest days of your life.'

Now, if you've got this far in this book, you'll know that these people were a bit careless regurgitating that trope in my direction. However, they were *kind of* right, in that my teenage years did still feature some of my happiest days, even in and amongst the traumatic times.

My years in sixth form were a back-and-forth of extremes. The loss hit me in a different way after that first anniversary – in a way where I started to miss him from my future. I started to long for his presence to accompany the rites of passage that come with 'coming of age', going from boy to man.

At school I started to knuckle down again. The disabled loo I mentioned earlier was still my place of refuge for in-school crying, but by sixth form this loo had a baby changing table facility added – a bizarre addition to a school toilet but nonetheless one I was grateful for. I'd often go in there, have a sob, get out my emotions and then place my laptop on the flap-down changing unit and use it as a TV table to watch the *EastEnders Omnibus*, all whilst sitting on the toilet lid and just having some time out.

I also made friends with the sixth-form receptionist, Annette, a tall, mid-to-late forties woman who wasn't a teacher but was just this incredibly sweet and clued-up adult. As soon as I started sixth form I would just chat to her, spending hours bitching about everything and anything that was annoying me. She became a real mentor for me that first year and I ended up getting three As and a B at AS level, beating any predictions that myself or the school had and so, soon enough, my head of sixth form told me that it would definitely be a good idea for me to apply to some universities.

As a child, this was something I had never really thought of as being in my future. No one in my family had ever gone. Not even in my extended family. Not even in my extended family's extended family. Going to uni was something I'd only ever heard of being slagged off down the pub as what lazy young poshos do to avoid doing any real work, and who then get paid more 'all because they've read some books!' There was a palpable working-class angst against student culture when I was growing up, one reflected in much of the comedy I remember watching at the time – stand-ups on *Live at the Apollo* all talking about students as lazy and lucky (as if they hadn't all been bloody Oxbridge candidates themselves!).

My dear nan, upon hearing that I may have a chance, became very vocal and desperate for me to go. If a grandson of hers had the opportunity to get a degree, she would strive to make it happen. So me, Nan and Mum agreed that, if I could get a maintenance grant and some financial help, then I should definitely pursue the chance.

The UCAS and careers advisor in my sixth orm centre met with me and asked me to think about what I'd like to do. The obvious choice to everyone was that I should study theatre and apply to some drama schools, but I really didn't want to. I always thought plays were really long and boring (still do now), I hated most musicals and, if I'm being totally honest, I just thought most drama-ery type students were really fucking annoying. It was all just bit too much for me. I loved acting and fiction and television, but I loved realism more. As a teenager, I felt that my experiences of grief had accelerated me straight into a level of adulthood that meant I couldn't be fucked to faff around with Brechtian acting techniques or experimental workshops where you'd pretend to be a dog for a day. I just wanted to tell stories about life and so I told my careers advisor: 'Journalism. I want to study journalism and become a proper journalist.'

I traipsed around numerous open days with my mum – a woman who had only ever stepped foot in a university to clean one. I knew the fancy red brick institutions and the prestige of Oxbridge would never be for me and that I wanted something vocational, creative and practical. Most of all, it was important that I stayed nearish home, near my mum, who was still struggling with Dad's loss. Thankfully, studying journalism meant the majority of good universities were all in London.

I decided to get some work experience to help my application and somehow I ended up meeting Radio 1 DJ Rob da Bank at a young person's workshop, all about how to start your own music festival – Rob co-founded Bestival. I went as part of my business studies coursework, where I created my own Glastonbury, but instead in a fairly shitty skatepark park in Watford, and I asked him if there were any media/press work experience opportunities. Rob said, 'No, but email me and I'll see what I can do.'

So I did. And two months later, in between Year 12 and 13, I was getting on the Isle of Wight ferry with my mum and her best mate, Rita, in a battered up Peugeot 203 and I'd been given a job as Rob da Bank's assistant's assistant at Bestival. Essentially, I was a very low-level event runner, being hands-on-deck to do anything I was asked, whenever it was needed.

This ended up including everything from getting the booze rider for my designated acts to actually driving my designated acts in a golf buggy to their stage set. And so I got La Roux eight bottles of Caribbean rum – they loved the stuff. Then I ran round all day being Rolf Harris's runner and sharing the last slice of lemon meringue pie in the artist catering tent with him, a story I told with utmost pride until we all found out he was a dodgy, sex-offending total bastard.

My final job was to drive a relatively unknown Janelle Monae and three trombonists to the Big Top stage for her performance. Once I'd dropped her off, an onsite manager asked me how I old I was, out of curiosity. I said sixteen and their face dropped. It turned out I was definitely too young and uninsured to be driving anyone around in a golf buggy, let alone Janelle Monáe. It was a truly bizarre set of jobs to be doing at sixteen, but everyone just presumed I was about twenty-four. I'd barely ever done a load of washing in my life by that point. It was a truly incredible weekend.

I wrote about the experience for our local magazine, who then asked me to be their youth reporter, working for a woman called Jill, who was like the Rita Skeeter of the outer-Watford villages. I'd put together articles on school issues or open mic nights or sometimes interview performers coming to a local venue, and my articles did quite well locally. Soon my psychology teacher Miss Glanville gave me a leaflet about the Roundhouse in Camden – an iconic music venue that secretly had an incredible creative workshop programme in little cave-like rooms underneath its mainstage. This programme taught teenagers from more challenging backgrounds everything from circus skills to music production and – most importantly for me – multimedia journalism.

I got on this year-long online magazine course and, soon enough, I was running around Camden Town every Wednesday night after school with a giant Dictaphone, getting vox pops from local residents, a unique mix of both posh Primrose Hill yummy mummies and friendly local drug dealers. Most of the time they were just telling me what they thought the London 2012 Olympics would be like.

I'd finish at the Roundhouse at 9pm, and my dad's best mate, Paul – who was also a black cab driver – would pick me up outside and we'd grab the same dodgy Chinese food from the same Camden Market stall that me and Dad used to frequent. Then Paul would drive me all the way back home to my mum's. Paul became like my confidant that year, and I knew our Wednesday night chats driving back home in his cab were helping him deal with my dad's loss as much as they were helping me. It was quite nice getting to know one of my dad's best mates for one hour every week as he drove me home and we shared some mini vegetable spring rolls. As I never ever spoke to my brothers about any of this grief for a very long time, I was so grateful that I had just one male presence in my life who was actively helping me. Who wanted me to make something of myself. Doing something Dad would be proud of.

After completing all these bits of work experience, I started to really throw myself into the idea of getting into university, because I knew it could be an escape. I saw it as potentially my way out from all the grief and constant reminders, and, a way to actually make my teenage years become the 'happiest ones of my life', like everyone said they should be.

And then, suddenly, came a gift. I had my first uni interview at the London College of Communication's journalism school and checked my UCAS portal a few days after to see I had been given an unconditional offer. They wanted me regardless of my A-level results, something quite rare back in 2010. Receptionist Annette and I started jumping up and down around the sixth-form office. I was the only one in my year to get such an offer, handed an actual place at an actual university and to be the first in my family to go.

This offer felt like a blessing, because it meant that the stress and pressure of my exams didn't need to consume me as much as they had been. I obviously wanted to do well, but I knew I had a back-up plan, and when an experience like grief strips you of back-up plans, this felt like karma. Like a real gift to be given some peace of mind that there was some sort of exciting, unknown future that might be waiting for me.

That evening, I told everyone around the kitchen table at dinner. My mum was elated. My brother's girlfriend stood up and gave me a hug. And Dean just sat picking at his plate and ignored it. He thought so poorly of students, seeing them as this lazy, work-shy stereotype, that he never said well done, something that nowadays I know he regrets.

When I knew that university was definitely on the cards, I started to stay back after school with Annette and search online for scholarship programmes, funding relief schemes and other ways to reduce the costs. I'd spend hours after hometime trawling through funding databases, filling in applications.

After weeks upon weeks of research, I came across a scholarship for a university with what I thought was the perfect course for me: BA Journalism, with a broadcast specialism. It was at a very central London university called the University of Westminster. The scholarship was a full £12,000 fee coverage, essentially meaning I wouldn't have to pay any tuition fees. It was incredible because it combined my dream to study in the media capital of the world with being affordable and close to my mum.

Then I read the small print – not about the scholarship, but the course itself. The campus was in Harrow. Harrow, which was a 15–20-minute Met Line train journey away. Harrow, which is exactly 11.9 miles away from my house. Harrow, where I'd had my tonsils out in the hospital next to the campus and where my brother Alan had done one of those dodgy but well-paid drugs trials, which got shut down after people started growing extra limbs! Bloody. Fucking. Harrow!

My mum was over the moon at the idea. The thought of me being so close still after all we'd been through, possibly on an all fees-paid scholarship, suddenly made it a desirable first option to follow.

So I applied.

The conditions of the scholarship were that you had to be from a means-tested household, you had to be the first in your family to go to university, you had to have a portfolio of work to show the department, you had to have experienced a personal hardship to show you were deserving and you had to have three As at A level. It was almost too good to be true. I had all but the latter going for me; I just needed to smash my exams, and I did, until my very last one.

My final examination was a two-hour English paper, where the fire alarm went off about 25 minutes in. We all got marched outside and my nerves fell to shit. I knew just how important it was that I got the results. It was worth £12k.

I remember thinking about what I could buy with £12k. I could buy anything with £12k! I could probably launch my own outlet of Wagamama with £12k. I tried to compose myself, but when I got back into the exam hall 15 minutes later, I felt like I'd frozen. Like I'd fucked it. You know that feeling in an exam when your brain just isn't even remotely focusing on the job at hand and the fear takes over? That was me. Right when I needed to be on my game. The exam finished and I wept and wept and wept. It was almost amazing that I was crying about an exam for once, because that felt like a normal thing to lose your shit over. That felt like a normal anxiety.

Results Day. Me and Mum walked into my sixth-form centre to get my results envelope. I opened it and burst into tears – again.

Three As.

After everything we'd been through, I'd done it. We'd done it. He'd done it. The reason I say 'he' – my dad – is because I noticed an asterisk next to my English A-level mark. My base-line exam score was actually two marks lower than an A, meaning I technically got a B. However, with the three-point mark-up you get for a 'distressing disruption' – such as a piercingly loud 15-minute-long fire alarm, my mark was boosted up one point into an A.

I got a £12,000 scholarship by one mark. One single mark.

And, to this day, I still believe, whether true or not, that a divine intervention from Dad set that fire alarm off.

I found out that my best mate Lewis had also got into the exact same university, same campus and everything, and so we would both be going together, which felt like the cherry on top of the cake.

We all celebrated by going down the Harvester with my aunties and cousins. I had four salad bowls, all smothered in celebratory red devil's sauce to render the health benefits of such salad useless. Did I have the bacon bits, fried onion shavings and the croutons? Of course I did, I'm not a monster!

I now had a chance, at eighteen years old, to get out of home. To be myself. To find out who I truly was beyond the boy whose dad died. I had a chance to get away and become myself again. (Even if it was only an 11.9 mile, 32-minute car drive and 24-minute Metropolitan Line train from my actual childhood house.)

big fat liar

When you are starting a new chapter for yourself, curating a new identity to introduce the new you to new people in a new area, you may very well find yourself lying through your teeth to make yourself seem 'not shit'.

Everyone to a certain extent revels in the opportunity to reinvent and almost upgrade oneself, whether you're chatting to some strange old bloke down the pub who you'll never see again or you're beginning a whole new life at the University of Westminster's Harrow Campus, specialising in media, art and design.

Examples of this particular reinvention may include adopting a nickname for yourself that no one has actually ever called you before – something like Dolly or Coco or just adding a -y to the end of your surname to appear notoriously fun. (Warning: anyone with a -y added to the end of their surname may not be notoriously fun at all, they may actually just be a bit of a douche.)

Perhaps you will pretend during a drinking game in freshers' week that you lost your virginity at a wild college house party, when really a guy called Pete (seventeen, acne sufferer) just prodded your genitals in an empty parental bedroom. Perhaps you might proclaim that you did ketamine for the first time in Year 9, so actually 'nothing ever fazes' you. Perhaps you might pretend you're closely related to Louis Theroux, like some lad did at my uni in a vain attempt to 'get pussy'. (We discovered he wasn't related to Louis Theroux when Louis Theroux came to our campus for a talk and didn't say hi to him.)

In a way, it seems somewhat imperative that fresh starts are fuelled by some lies, just to help present yourself as better than your averages, to use a self-invented mythology to 'jujge' or 'zhuzh' up your relatively normal life and attract cool people.[1] It's the identity equivalent of sticking chicken fillets in your bra or filtering all your selfies to death – it's not necessarily representative of the truth, but it might be the lil' confidence boost that helps you somehow feel *more* like you.

Sadly, my fibbing began before I even started my course and now, after eight years, I feel it is time to divulge my deceptive misdemeanours and admit that … I lied (*sort of*) to get into my university.[2]

---

[1]   Fuck knows if it's spelt 'jujge', 'zhuzh' or 'tszuj'. It's a truly stupid word. I did a Twitter poll to see how people spelt it and the first two options came out equally on top.

[2]   You can lock me up like Lynette from *Desperate Housewives* (the real-life actor was caught sneakily paying for her daughter to get into an elite US college) and then you can put me in a goddamn prison boiler suit (which are actually very slimming on me), because I am a big fat fucking liar.

My home address was within a 25-mile radius of my campus, so unfortunately, by the rules, I was not eligible for a room in my university's halls of residence. This worried me, because I knew that university had to be, in a way, an escape from those past three years of grief – a way of physically moving on from a warm, loving home that I cherished dearly, but that had also contained so much pain and heartache. For my advancement, for my survival almost, I needed to get out and so I concocted a really quite convincing and unprovable lie.

Upon accepting my university offer in August, I rang up this woman called Karen on the Accommodation and Student Housing Team (they're always called Karen) and I told her that my mum was moving to Canada. I convincingly droned on about how my departure signalled the time for my mum to up sticks and start a new life – which she was hastily planning to do before Christmas, so I urgently needed to secure housing ASAP. To seal the deal of this lie, I emotionally waxed lyrical to Kaz about how my beloved dad had traumatically died three years before and now that I was considered an adult by the state, my widowed mother was off on this fresh Canadian start, with waffles and pine trees and maple syrup and ... whatever else is Canadian ... ?

I don't know why I chose Canada, perhaps I just thought it was the friendliest country who'd openly take in widows from all over the shop to move in to nice quaint box-towns in Quebec. I had watched this exact storyline in nearly every single 'true movie' that my mum used to watch on the shit film channels you get lurking about on Sky+. Those sort of strange, US-heavy content networks that loom around the channel 320–340 mark, which just schedule TV movie after TV movie where a newly single woman starts a new life in a new town and meets a strapping fifty-something carpenter named Brock.

In all these films, Brock is incidentally also widowed/divorced/sinisterly single and by coincidence is living right next door to newly single woman! Brock is always depicted as 'salt 'n' pepper' handsome, only ever wearing plaid shirts, in which he often chops down big trees, suffering with the weight of his own silent masculinity. Naturally, he owns a golden Labrador – his only real companion in life and a dog who likely watches him cry-wank each night with a bottle of ice-cold Budweiser out the mini-fridge of his hand-built, timber-framed man cave. Then, after months of passive flirtation across pine-tree-lined streets, Brock, the newly single woman and the golden lab all start their own family together, shacking up and walking about Canadian forests or along Canadian beaches or around Canadian lakes, before going home to put up a Canadian Christmas tree and enjoy spoonful upon spoonful of Canadian maple syrup. Dreamy.

Sometimes I wish my mum had actually moved to this dreamlike, fictional vision of Canada avec Brock, but alas my phone call with Karen was just a lie to get me bumped up to the priority student housing list. And through manipulating Karen's sympathy towards my recently deceased father – and despite the likelihood that she too may have watched many of these hammed-up emotional 'true movies' – my lie managed to work.

That week I was offered a room in halls, given a move-in date and Student Finance England sorted out the rest. Lewis was so jealous, as he was going to remain at home and just commute in every day, but I promised he could just crash at mine whenever.

I told my mum that, if she were asked by my university on move-in day about her expatriation to the North American Commonwealth, she was to recite some tripe about her upcoming new life with Brock, and then next year we could just claim Brock was a toy boy trying to steal all Mum's money, like all the blokes in *Take a Break* magazine always seem to do, thus Canada fell through. It was the perfect lie.

And it was one ... of many. Two.

moving-in day

September 2011

We packed Aunty Jenny's Ford estate full of all my shit, including: random DVDs like *Scooby-Doo 2: Monsters Unleashed* that I had neither any intention to ever watch again nor a DVD player on which to do so; books that were too juvenile for me to ever want to read again; and a childhood Junior Scrabble board that I would never play with again but which would later play host to numerous lines of coke, snorted during a halls party that I wasn't actually present for.

It was a strange ceremony, boxing up my adolescence, almost feeling like a funeral for my childhood and a reminder of past days where everything seemed innocent. Where I felt naive and carefree. (Only someone coming from real sheltered happiness could ever endure the flimsy plot of *Scooby Doo 2* for 98 minutes anyway.)

157

After three hours of packing, Jenny, Josie and I set off on the trepidatious 11.9-mile car drive to my halls of residence. Despite the proximity, I could sense my mum's intense nerves at the prospect of me leaving – we had been such an unstoppable, solid team for those past three years. It must have been like when Dec got the plane to Australia in 2018 to host *I'm a Celebrity ... Get Me Out of Here!* without Ant, because Ant was having an *annus horribilis*.

It felt like things would never be the same again. But Josie slapped on a brave face, forgot to apply waterproof mascara and we all drove on to the A404 with shit Costa Express lattes from the petrol garage to toast my new beginning. My new chapter was as much a new one for her as it was for me.

As always, my Aunty Jenny's car was soundtracked by low-volume Radio 4 mutterings. The station was doing a ten-year memorial programme to the victims of the 9/11 attacks.

'A mass murder of 3,000 innocent, working civilians,' droned on in the background of an already tense car journey. Mum silently stared out the window as Aunty Jenny incessantly went on about how I should strategically make friends with other freshers.

'Maybe invite them into your room for a cuppa or see if they want to bake cakes, or perhaps ask if they'd like to go to the big Sainsbury's with you? You can all do your shopping together! God it's exciting! I wish I was off to university,' she exclaimed, whilst Mum slapped the scan button on the car stereo.

We really didn't need this beginning of the new chapter of our lives to be scored by the harrowing testimonials of

9/11 survivors. The radio landed on Capital FM and instead we listened yet again to Adele's 'Someone Like You', which at this period in time felt like it had been number one for an eternity.

'Don't forget me, I beg,' Mum sang, looking back at my face, a half-joking, half-serious reminder that she still needed me around. Little did she know I'd stick quite rigidly to my promise of coming home at least every fortnight to see her, mainly with a whole suitcase full of dirty washing and a desire to raid the vegetable section of her fridge – a section I'd rarely frequented when I was a permanent child resident.

As we pulled up to my campus for the first time, it was the usual scene of a student halls move-in. Boot doors pointed skywards, with teenage crap spilling out the back of ubiquitous family cars. Mums and dads and siblings and dogs all congregated around their precious eighteen/nineteen-year-old, about to leave the comforting bosom of their family home for shit shags, drunken fingering, over-priced lectures and pre-drinks at Georgia's before going to Oceania in Watford.

As we opened our car boot I saw my Aunty Jenny touch my mum's arm – a reassurance that it was all going to be OK. Perhaps it was an arm touch that my dad would have given my mum if we were one of these normal 2.4 nuclear families. Perhaps it was a token of 'He'll be OK, Josie.' And yet, in my mad, paranoid teenage mind, perhaps low-key knowing that these university years would be the forum where I'd explore some of the very confusing same-sex attractions that had been racing through my head, I suddenly thought: WHAT

IF EVERYONE THINKS I HAVE LESBIAN MUMS! WHAT DOES THIS PUBLIC ARM TOUCH SUGGEST?! I've enough on my plate without being the boy with ruddy lesbian mums!

Just to remind you that this was September 2011. This was pre-woke queer awareness era. I was eighteen and, if you'd have asked me what 'LGBT' meant, I would have said a sandwich. I was definitely still struggling with an acute but consistently present level of internalised homophobia. Freshly turned eighteen-year-old me still described things that were crap as 'gay', like many other teenagers my age.

Nowadays, as a man who mostly trusts the judgement of my queer female friends, I would *fucking kill to have lesbian mums*. What an absolute blessing it would be. Imagine how well dressed you'd be as a toddler – in durable, sustainable, yet perfectly colour-matched fashion. Yes, please!

So, in that moment, on the ten-year anniversary of 9/11, stood outside a block of new-build university halls in South Harrow, I read too much into this token of sisterly affection and it triggered my already growing anxieties: I just did not want to draw attention to myself as 'different' at uni. I felt so strongly that this new chapter was a chance for reinvention – not in the pretentious name-changing way, but in that of no longer feeling like the boy whose dad died. Of no longer being someone whose family were a point of local gossip or discussion, no matter how well-intentioned. I wanted to at last be normal. A normal eighteen-year-old teenager.

And so, in that halls car park, I pathetically made a real point of persistently and loudly referring to Jenny as 'AUNTY JENNY!' and my mum as 'MUM'.

Obviously no one picked up on this whatsoever and no one gave a fuck.

As AUNTY! Jenny unpacked the boot, Mum and I went to pick up the keys and entry card to my accommodation from Karen in reception, who fortunately never mentioned my mum's upcoming 'move to Canada'. I was assigned a room in Flat 83, a fourteen-bedroom, soon-to-be party flat in the premium block, right next to the main entrance on the ground floor. Mum wasn't happy about that, because she thought it increased my chances of getting robbed. I was *very* happy about it because it decreased my chances of ever climbing stairs.

There was, however, one more 'white' lie that I tried out on poor Karen.

Since the age of six, I had always slept in a double bed – a measure implemented by my dad, as I'd nightly roll out of my childhood single bed whilst asleep and terrify myself awake through falling two foot to the ground. Dad got fed up of me screaming myself awake at 3.30am and so bought me a double bed with a wooden surround to prevent me chucking myself out. This was then my bed for twelve years and I eventually grew out of my sleepy-fish bowl suicide tendencies.

Now, a decade later, the prospect of sleeping daily in a single halls bed frame felt like a downgrade I must strive to prevent, especially considering the premium block rooms could easily fit a double, so I concocted another lie. I told Karen that I had Willis-Ekbom disorder, more popularly known as restless legs syndrome. It's a common condition that causes an overwhelming and irresistible urge to move one's legs, and is mostly associated with involuntary leg jerking during sleep.

So I asked Karen if I could have a double bed. For my condition. She sweetly exclaimed, 'Oh, honey, we don't have any double beds, my sweetheart.' This was a woman who BARELY knew me, but spoke in a tone of voice so passionate I felt like she'd fight for my life.

'But I do have a plan for you, hun.'

I think Karen must have thought, poor fucker – he's just lost his dad, his mum's fucking off to Canada and he's got a neurological disorder that prevents him having a good night's kip. So she called the caretakers, and as me, Mum and AUNTY! Jenny were moving all my crap into my halls room, a handy-man knocked on the door and delivered a second single bed, courtesy of Karen. This eventually had a double mattress slapped on top to give me what was to be infamously known as 'the most comfortable bed in halls', whilst also being big enough to have the best sex a fresher could ever wish for in halls. No one should have to have sex in a single bed, yet everyone was supposed to. The saddest part of this story is that I did not *once* have sex in this bed.

At last, all my stuff was out the car and the time came for them to leave. Aunty Jenny hugged me, reminding me that she lived approximately a 14-minute tube journey away while squeezing me so tight it was as if I'd moved to the University of Aberystwyth. She went out to the car and left me and my mum to say farewell. I don't think we actually said anything. She was too strong to break down in front of me. I reassured her that I would be OK, that the main reason I was at this university was not only that my fees were paid for, but also so I could still be close to her. She nodded, smiled, kissed my forehead, chimed out her catchphrase of 'Be safe!' and headed out to the car park. I sat by the window and waved them goodbye as they drove off and left.

I sat on my bed, soaking up the silence. I didn't feel abandoned or like I'd been pushed into university. This was exactly what I wanted for my future. I just felt so gutted that this future didn't have my dad looking after my mum as I moved out and grew up into an adult man. Who would look after her? And so I did something I had never done before.

I prayed.

I pulled together the paper-thin blue curtains of my halls room, got down on two knees at my bedside and prayed. I prayed to Dad to make sure she would be OK. To make sure I would be OK.

And then, once these prayers were over, I sat back on my bed and downloaded Grindr. I had been waiting to do this ever since I heard comedians cracking jokes about it and so, on this momentous day, I put the app on to my HTC android phone for the very first time.[1] I didn't even open the app

---

[1]   Any millennial homosexual male will tell you how you will almost certainly delete the Grindr app ten times in distress and then eventually re-download it. You may last months without it, maybe weeks. I once downloaded it literally an hour after deletion. I am pathetic. Alas, this deletion phenomenon is now sadly a part of the rite of passage of being a twenty-first-century gay.

for weeks and weeks after this. I just kept it on my phone, hidden in a faraway folder. Knowing it was something I eventually needed to address.

Fifteen minutes later my Aunty Jenny called.

'Hiya, Jack, I think I've gone and left my house keys on your shelf!'

Before I knew it they were both back in my room with Wenzel's bakery bags full of sausage rolls and egg mayo sandwiches, Mum covered in tear-trailed mascara after crying almost immediately after turning on to the A404 back home.

'I'm fucking gutted, babe,' she sobbed. 'It feels like my fucking heart's been fucking ripped out!', which is probably what you, dearest reader, would also say if I moved out of your house too!

Jenny and Mum stayed for another hour and we met a few of my flatmates. I think it helped my mum to realise that there were thirteen other people going through this too. Thirteen other people who were as scared and anxious and nervous. And whilst those others hadn't been through what we had been through for those past few years of grief, I think my mum realised that this was the best way for me to regain some of my childhood. Some of my youth. Some of my innocence.

Second time lucky, they eventually left. This was it.

how to support someone who you're leaving behind

1 Remind them that, although you've gone, you're still always there for them.

2 Arrange a specific time to speak – and try your hardest not to move or cancel. Make it a priority call that you can both look forward to. Something regular to stay in contact.

3 Put a date in the diary for a catch-up, the next dinner or trip out somewhere. Be organised so you can spend quality time together.

4 Put the effort in. This sounds obvious, but it can be hard when you've moved somewhere new to find that time and energy. But you also never quite know how speaking to someone from home, someone familiar and who knows you, who loves you regardless and is going to remind you of how proud they are of you, can actually really help with how you may be feeling. It can often be a pick-me-up you didn't even know you needed. I often try to do this with my friends who I know have been through shit times and have come out the other side. And it doesn't matter how much geographical or time distance may exist between you, you can always remind someone of what they mean to you.

5 Lastly – don't beat yourself up too much. It is hard to stay in touch with people. These things are always presented as easy, but if your energy is being directed in lots of new directions, just say that. Moving on from one chapter to the next is all about compromise and balance. Make sure you're clear what you can and can't do with someone who might be missing you, and then make sure when you spend that time with them that you are fully focused on them.

flat 83

Fourteen students in one halls flat is an intimidating amount of people, personalities and personal kitchenware to respect and live side by side with. Imagine S Club 7 and then times it by two!

The bunch of characters in Flat 83 included but was not limited to:

The classic stoner illustrator adorned with incredible tattoos, hailing from a northern city, which gave her a comfortingly similar tone of voice to Lauren Laverne.

The camp fashion student who'd leave passive-aggressive Post-its on his humous pot.

An incredibly kind girl from Sussex who always had a hotel reception bowl of Ferrero Rochers, peppered with Rafaellos and various flavours of Lindt choccy balls, by the door of her room. She would share these with any visitor because she was so lovely.

The proud socialist who'd use the kitchen table as his propaganda soapbox.

The token Tory who was completely out of her depth on a creative liberal campus.

A French girl who'd speak so intensely close to your face that you felt like she was about to nut you at any given moment.

An older mature student who had a two-door Alfa Romeo parked outside the flat and would drive anyone at any time to the 24-hour Asda superstore in Wembley Park to procure post-spliff munchies, Dairylea Lunchables, a milk carton full of highly concentrated tropical fruit juice or sometimes even just someone's weekly shop.

And last but not least, a gym addict, who I sadly believe is likely to experience arthritis later in life from the grip that his hands had on a 750ml protein shake bottle, clasped so tightly as he marched to the gym each morning that you'd think it contained his mother's ashes.

Everyone, on the whole, in Flat 83 was pretty lovely; I felt I had truly lucked out and we spent nine months together in relative bliss, except for one girl who we all suspected was perhaps night-time pissing into empty two-litre Lilt bottles whilst in bed and then pouring said piss out of her bedside window, despite all of us being in rooms with EN SUITE TOILETS!

One time a flatmate expressed this personal (collective) paranoia that she poured piss out the windows and piss girl went absolutely ballistic. Doors were slammed. Food was stolen. The energy in the flat turned to one of shame, because what if she didn't pour piss out the window? The outstanding evidence was that the external wall and window sill of her room, which were mainly where people would congregate to pass around a spliff, always stunk like a urinal at an all boys' school. But what if that was just by chance? What if some weird second year, longing for their fresher year, kept urinating against the window of their old halls room in a bizarre mark of territory? We'll never know. I tried my hardest to still be nice, because you never know what sort of troubles a window-pisser is going through – you really can't have had an easy life if you're pouring piss out a window. However, she then moved out and was replaced by an Italian student who was so rich that he never washed his clothes, he just bought more and more and more new ones. It was absolutely astonishing. I quite missed the window-pisser.

The first few weeks of term involved everyone chumming up quite intensely. Friendships and alliances were quickly forged, perhaps out of anxiety and a fear of the unknown three years that lay ahead of us. Soon enough, the term BFFL was being banded around on Facebook photo captions as casually as chlamydia in the hotel rooms of central Magaluf.

At this time, I distinctly remember that I pissed off some of my school friends by so quickly becoming immersed in how much I loved all my flatmates. Some of my school friends detested theirs, complaining of feeling lonely and out of place. Meanwhile, I was jovially stealing Sainsbury's trolleys with mine, getting fucked on Corky's Strawberry-and-Cream liquor shots and speeding down our halls car park with three in a cart. It was all so much fun.

Some of you will relate to this and some of you may have never experienced it, but after the three years I'd had, those three weeks of freshers were exactly what I'd needed. Pure silly fun. Running along halls corridors into other people's kitchen parties, meeting all sorts of characters – like what I imagine it would have been to attend boarding school or Hogwarts.

I remember my flatmate Steph inviting me to go round to some of her course-mates' kitchen for a little soiree. She was studying fine art and illustration, so everyone on her course was terribly creative and abstract in an intimidatingly fun way. And with ten of us sat sharing some horrendously strong home-made punch that had been poured into one big central bowl, soon came a rite of passage for any fresher – the game of the twenty-first century: Never Have I Ever.

The premise being that you would say something outrageous that you'd 'never done' and then you'd see who in the room had done it if they took a swig of their drink. However, in this version of the game it was flipped, so everyone would say the most outrageous thing they had done in order to show off, *and* take a swig. This way the game was designed to get everyone absolutely trashed as soon as possible.

The demographic of this game was seven boys, three girls, ten cups. We went round one by one.

'Never Have I Ever taken amphetamines,' cracked the voice of a Scouse girl.

'Never Have I Ever had sex on my period,' said the next, the pair of them swigging.

'Never Have I Ever tasted my own cum!' proudly announced a very sweet guy who was a part-time drag queen at the weekends.

These got extreme quite quickly for a bunch of relatively nuanced visual art students. And as they were coming thick and fast, my turn was approaching. What could I say that made me seem fun and self-deprecating? Something that was universal yet unique. And so I sat up and proudly exclaimed, 'Never Have I Ever shat myself!'

I drank because, sadly, I have on a few upsetting occasions committed such a terrible crime. Only one other person drank, another lad called Jack. We smiled.

'It's horrible, isn't it?' he said. I nodded profusely.

After sharing our stories of self-shitting, up came the next batch of Nevers.

'Never Have I Ever been tied up.'

'Never Have I Ever given a cab driver a blowjob.'

'Never Have I Ever been fucked whilst dressed in leather.'

A few more people took swigs at each admission and Steph started going round, topping up everyone's cups with more of the poisonous punch via an IKEA ladle from one of those student starter utensils multipacks. My cup didn't need topping up because I had basically done NONE of these things.

One of the other boys called Louis – who I'd clocked straight away because he was beardy and clearly gay – leaned in to the group and said: 'Never Have I Ever shagged someone of the same sex.'

And all of a sudden everyone drank apart from me and Jack. We smiled at each other again. Everyone laughed.

'Well Jack and Jack should shag now!' shouted Steph. Jack laughed and so I laughed, however I totally would have been down for it if I had even possessed a shred of confidence. That and also Jack was most certainly straight. This was confirmed by the fact his girlfriend was actually sat next to him.

Now, I should have used this opportunity to say something cheeky and honest like 'I haven't slept with a guy but I really want to!' I was in the safest possible space to say that. But I was almost quite relieved to be presented so quickly as straight. I was relieved to be given the presumption of heterosexuality. And so, with that internal shame kept firmly to myself, I decided to strike up a chat with the other Jack.

His surname was Groves, so we agreed upon Spice Girls-esque distinctions of Jack G and Jack R. Jack G was very sweet, a relatively shy lad from near Brighton. Somehow knowing he was from the queer capital of England made me feel quite at ease and his relaxed demeanour in a room mostly full of queer men was refreshing. He was kind, silly, up for a laugh. He told me that his best friend was on my course, a guy called Brendan, whom he had been to college with.

Steph shouted across the room, 'Oh, is that the lad who's on that new Channel 4 documentary?'

Jack G nodded.

It conspired that this Brendan guy was taking part in a series called *Living with the Amish*, where a set of British teenagers, on a spectrum of bratty to bizarre, headed to the

States for six weeks to live amongst the infamous traditionalist Christians. Brendan was the 'cool, nerdy, BlackBerry-obsessed' typecast. The press that the programme received depicted him as a trendy, indie Brighton boy. Everyone on campus knew who he was because the show was airing just as we were starting uni.

Soon Brendan was on *Heat* magazine's 'Man-O-Meter', placed right at the very top as the hottest guy of the week and he was shagging seemingly every girl I'd met on campus. I'd had one brief chat with him and, guess what? I hated him.

I hated him in that immature eighteen-year-old kind of way, like writing someone off because they didn't enjoy the same bands as you. He had done nothing bad to me, except one of his Facebook photos was a photo of him in the Rough Trade photo booth and that felt like a crime of sorts.

Looking back, I probably found Brendan intimidating and I was also probably jealous. (I was definitely jealous.)

free shit

The University of Westminster freshers' fair was like a meat market, full of horny, petrified eighteen/nineteen-year-olds figuring out what they can do for three years aside from make pesto pasta and masturbate.

There was a line of stalls, which each represented either a specialist leisure activity, such as football, American football, netball, basketball, handball and even more exciting games involving balls, or a commercial venture – spunking out free promotional material to excitable students who were all horny for as much free shit as possible.

You could get absolutely buzzing off numerous free cans of Monster energy drink before doing the Nando's spicy wing roulette challenge, thanks to some poor sod who was roaming around campus in a full-sized Portuguese chicken costume giving out free vouchers. Then you could go round filling up a tote bag with infinite supplies of free pens, keyrings, bottle openers, bottle openers which doubled up as keyrings, Oyster card holders I'd never use, condoms (I'd never use, not out of choice but lack of chance), lollipops, rain ponchos and a DIY STI kit to help tackle campus chlamydia rates.

It was promotions heaven and, looking back, the amount of single-use plastic would have given Greta Thunberg a mild panic attack. How many people even use a fucking Oyster-card holder?

Walking in and amongst the freshers at the fair were puffa jacket-wearing second years, otherwise known as 'the campus drug dealers', who were also doing the rounds to find new clientele for the academic year. They identified their potential customers very cleverly through clothing choices and haircut types and somehow they absolutely nailed it. They knew the fashion students wanted coke and the music students wanted weed and the visual arts students wanted pretty much anything they could get their hands on, and they catered for them very well.

As I walked round, the first people I bumped into were Jack Groves and his friend Brendan, Brendan somehow capturing the attention of cool guys (aka, the boys I fancied) and cool girls (aka, the girls I wanted to be friends with). He was what would be considered a BNOC (Big Name on Campus), an indie lad in skinny jeans with a scruffy haircut who could have easily fallen out the pages of *NME* magazine. Upon seeing him and Jack G, rather than maturely say hello, I just looked down and picked up an HSBC student account Oyster-card holder.

At the fair, I also saw Lewis looking around with all his photography course pals. It was weird bumping into him around our university – my best friend for nearly twenty years also bombing about the same corridors but with a whole other clique of friends from a different course. I think we silently yet defiantly made a concerted effort in that first term of university to have some distance, some separation in order to court other friends – a bit like a relationship on a break or us opening up to more partners. I think, as I was so quickly thrust into a world where I was being constantly confronted with an intense culture of sexuality, shagging and the gossip-filled discussions of 'who do you have your eye on?', it felt important to have some distance from Lewis. I was so closeted that, if I was to try to open that closet, it needed to be in the fresh arms of new friends and new people, even though I knew he would never have judged me, so an appropriate amount of distance was kept between us.

And it was at this freshers' fair that I met two very important people in the development of my life, who in many ways have affected my character, personality and the direction my adult life has taken.

First up – a guy called Nick Mathieson, who was also studying journalism. I fancied Nick immediately. He was fit, a bit stubbly, three years older than all of us and he had a gentle sort of bravado about him. Just a slightly more confident persona that probably came with age. He was a bit of a lad, loved football and was also really ambitious. I knew he was straight but I had a crush on him. He kept hanging around with a girl called Georgia on our course, who was a definite 10/10 and who I really liked. They were always arm-in-arm, flirtatiously laughing. They looked like a couple. They looked like everything I wished I was during freshers' week – hot, horny and heterosexually inclined.

As course-mates, Nick and I had politely nodded to each other, and I'd managed to keep my tongue from touching his non-consensually in the process. But we first spoke during the freshers' fair when I watched him walk up to the student radio station stall. I was stood just behind him.

The only student society I had any remote interest in was our university's radio station, SMOKE Radio. It was the one thing on the open day that I'd become excited at trying out. I knew that most of the current crop of Radio 1 DJs had all emerged from the often cringey world of university broadcasting and I couldn't wait to get a slice of that audio-content pie.

UK student radio is comprised of a bizarre mix of personnel: audio techie geeks who live life at a constant level of passive aggression; wannabe famous presenters who invariably adopt an annoying local radio voice any time they're in front of a mic; music nerds who love Belle and Sebastian and want an hour show to play their unique brand of off-kilter electronica-meets-jazz-infused-disco-meets-nu-wave-minimalist-broken-beat-ska-meets-Americana-indie music. There was a very weird bunch of characters, and once I started working in radio after university, I realised that these stereotypes didn't fade out. They are just as present in the professional world and I am a strange combination of all three. My dream job is still to have my own specialist music show on BBC 6 Music where I just play a lot of queer music for 90 minutes and ask Kathy Burke to do the news.

The student radio station, SMOKE, was run by a committee of elected second years. Station manager Natalie was a slightly older student who Nick charmed into giving him a show in remarkably fast fashion.

Then there was Jimmy, who ran the music playlists and was soon swarmed by lots of boys in hoodies with left hoop earrings begging for that specialist music programme I just described.

And then, finally, there was a guy called Olly, who was the head of news for the station. I approached him and said hello.

The first thing he said back was: 'Is that a wig?'

'Er no, it's my actual hair.'

'Mate, your haircut is fucking stupid.'

As you can see from the front cover of this book, I'm inclined to say he was and still is mildly right, but, nonetheless, I had made a first impression as I tried to convince him to give me a radio show. Once he'd touched my hair and believed I'd grown it myself, I told Olly how I wanted to do a magazine-style radio show, something that still contained music but was about news stories and social issues that affected the student body. He was mildly interested and told me to apply with a pitch and they'd get back to me soon. I didn't hold out too much hope.

On my way out of the freshers' fair, I remember walking past the LGBTQ+ society and looking at their stall. They were all unashamedly queer, wearing slogan T-shirts that at the time I felt were either a bit too long or a bit too short for my liking. They wore oversized jewellery and had amazing posture. They didn't look like 'my people', they looked amazing. I walked past thinking, 'Nah, not for me.' With hindsight, I am so upset I did that. I wish I had been braver. I wish I hadn't written them off and had instead tried to forge alliances. It would have made everything much, much easier.

pre-drinks

Before I arrived at uni, my drink of choice had always been cider. Lager was too grainy and bitter for me and I longed for the sweet crisp apple taste of shit, pissy White Lightning. I was a two-litre bottle of Strongbow tucked away in a cupboard kinda gal, with an accompanying bottle of Sainsbury's own double-concentrated blackcurrant squash at the ready, to snakebite and sugar up my drink to increase my consumption. Every now and then I'd treat myself to three mixed berry Kopparbergs for £5 from the big Sainsbury's. However, 2011 was the year that I was introduced to my now ex-best friend … white Zinfandel rose.

White Zinfandel rose wine came storming into my life like a runaway train. They were mostly priced around £5 a bottle and they got me much drunker, much quicker and with less of a tendency to cause me to burp or wee every 15 minutes. Soon enough I was in a monogamous relationship with white Zinfandel. The cider bottles appeared in my shopping trolley less and less. Instead, white Zinfandels would worm their way in, from the cheap brands of Gallo

Family and Blossom Hill to the occasional premium bottles of Beringer Blush – which still only had a £2 price differential in Saino's. It was just such a cheap way to get fucked.

Whether you called it 'pre-drinks' or 'pre-lash' became a sign of your own personal integrity and probable social class. 'Lash' tended to stem from posh boys entrenched in masculine bravado, who saw drinking as one of many competitive sports they engaged with, whereas I was much more of a 'pre-drinks' kinda gal. I still cringe at the term today.

'Pre-drinks' would happen in one of my friend's kitchens, on a rotational basis, whether that was Georgia in Flat 29, Alex in Flat 18 or mine at Flat 83. It would involve predominantly sitting or standing around a breakfast bar with your own plastic bag full of booze. You'd be listening to someone's Spotify playlist and then having to turn off frequent Purina Cat adverts blasting out in between Destiny's Child 'Lose My Breath' and Amerie's '1 Thing' – two songs which deserve a place in the pre-drinkers hall of fame. True bangers either before, during or after a night out.

The final thing to know about 'pre-drinks' is that you would only ever leave 'pre-drinks' once you'd downed all the contents of your own plastic bag of booze. I'd often stare at Nick downing cans of Foster's whilst I was drinking white Zinfandel out the bottle with a straw. And then, once considerably pissed, everyone would leave in a pack, often minus one or two characters who'd peaked too soon and were 'chundering' (that's posh people language for vomiting) in someone's en suite loo.

Then a collective drunken pilgrimage began to one iconic event on the University of Westminster's Harrow campus, a student night forever etched into my memory so much so that I can smell it anytime I walk past a pub's bins ... Messi Mondayz!

messi mondayz

October–November 2011

Messi Mondayz was horrifically spelt with an 'i' and a 'z'. It was a club night that saw the full length and breadth of student self-destruction. Shit UK Top 40 music, cheap booze, sticky dance floors – you know the night.

It took place at the Undercroft bar, a basement social space far too small for everyone to fit in with a dilapidated garden/smoking area, a tiny dance floor, some tatty snooker tables and a bar that proudly displayed sweaty Rollover hotdogs, stale un-toasted paninis and Sahara hot nuts. (Do you remember Sahara hot nuts? They were crunchy coated peanuts served warm. I *LOVED* Sahara hot nuts.)

The themes of Messi Mondayz during the first term would vary. There was the school disco party, where you'd dress up as slutty versions of the children you were only about four years before. There was the traffic light party, where, if you were taken, you dressed in red, if you were frigid you dressed in orange and if you were either of those options or single, you dressed in green ... I cannot stress this enough: EVERYONE DRESSED IN GREEN! Some boys even painted their skin green so as to indicate how much they wanted to fuck! It was all a bit much.

Everything was about fucking or geared around fucking and that fucking was always about boys fucking girls and girls getting fucked by boys. And I still wasn't sure who I wanted to fuck. I was too scared to approach any boys.

At one particular Messi Mondayz night a couple of months into my first year, I remember seeing handsome Nick Mathieson and Georgia dancing together, and I stared, just watching him. His mannerisms when he danced were almost quite camp. Most straight lads at my university would dance either by swaying with their arms around each other as if celebrating at an FA cup final, or jumping up and down in unison as if celebrating a goal being scored at an FA cup final. Whereas Nick was using his hands, gesticulating, dancing with not just Georgia but a few girls. I saw him as quite a ladies' man.

At this time, it was very on-trend to be a ladies' man. I went to university during the era of Psy's 'Gangnam Style', Robin Thicke's 'Blurred Lines' and certain types of boys in Abercrombie & Fitch shirts, collars popped up, leering at girls in short skirts. This was just before a new wave of student-accessible feminism in 2013/14 tried to wash all the muckiness away, or at least make more young men aware of their actions towards women.

On this one night, for some reason, everyone ended up back in my kitchen after Messi Mondayz. Georgia came in my room with me and we sat on my bed drinking secret reserves of white Zinfandel that I'd stashed away. It was very foolish to leave any precious perishables in the halls kitchen, so I'd often hide anything of alcoholic or snack importance floating in some cold water in my en-suite sink basin.

In a haze of drunkeness, I told Georgia, 'I think I might be bisexual ... '

She very sweetly held my hand and told me that was totally fine. She explained how that was what university was all about. And all of a sudden, streams of tears just erupted out of me and I told her everything. About my teenage years, about my dad, about my mum, about how much I was actually really missing home even though I was a mere 11.9 miles away. Georgia very sweetly hugged me and promised everything would be OK. We sat on my bed, silently passing the Zinfandel bottle back and forth to each other.

'You and Nick make a nice couple,' I said.

Georgia drunkenly chuckled.

'Have you been dating?' I asked.

She looked at me and laughed. 'No! Nick's gay!'

'Nick's not gay!' I retorted.

'Of course Nick's gay!'

In this moment a surge of excitement rushed from my stomach to my face and I couldn't help but beam with a feeling of underlying joy. There was actually someone in my extended uni friendship group who was both homosexual and who I had a crush on. And, yes, I thought he was totally out of my league, but that didn't matter ... he was a gay.

She told me how he was not publicly or openly out, but that most of his friends at university already knew. He had been pulling lads on campus, she said, and that as he's twenty-one and a bit older than us, he's been having sex with guys for a few years. It was all one big revelation, one that she could see, written all over my face, had excited me.

'Do you fancy Nick!? You fancy Nick! Don't you?!' she chanted, shortly before running from my bed to be sick in my sink. She didn't make it to the toilet bowl in time and was subsequently sick all over my Sainsbury's Be Good to Yourself Moroccan humous. I surprisingly didn't mind, despite that being my most premium regular purchase at the time.

This was all a magical moment of sorts. I admitted my crush and we agreed I should try to get to know Nick better. That I needed to confide in and speak to an actual gay person.

Georgia continued to be sick into the early hours and so we resigned ourselves to bed, instead choosing to watch *Gavin & Stacey* series one until 4am and riding out our morning hangover by bingeing series two. Cracking.

the first six months of being a gay

December 2011–May 2012

Your first love is a long-awaited rite of passage, culturally depicted in almost every coming-of-age film and half-baked BBC Three teen drama. The first kiss, the first time you say 'I love you', the trials and tribulations of that first intimate moment where you make love with someone you've waited a two-decade 'lifetime' to find. Everything's built up and aggrandised, but the reality is never an auspicious moment of first love and that first person you fall for may likely be a bit of a cunt.

Let's just remember that there is someone in this world who's first love was Bashar al-Assad or worse, Nasty Nick from *Big Brother* series one, and I say let's pray for them!

Many first loves turn out to be heartbreakers handing you your first slice of rejection. For me this ended up being – Nick Mathieson.

As soon as I'd found out Nick was gay, I started lingering around him just that bit too long, like a bad-smelling bin or a sexist uncle that doesn't know when to go home on Christmas Day. I began to put myself in places where I knew he'd be: the student union bar, the Junction pub in Harrow, the silent zone of the library – a pointless place to follow someone into when you're desperate to burst out feelings of being a closeted homosexual.

I began to just place myself around his periphery, trying to become better friends so I could eventually have someone gay to come out to and hopefully get some semblance of support from. However, the importance I was placing on this, combined with the sheer levels of internalised shame I had placed on myself, meant I was becoming more and more besotted with Nick, often to the point of jeopardising sane behaviour.

I started going weekly to the absolute cringe fest that was Yates Bar karaoke night in Harrow. Yates was a sports bar on the high street, mainly populated by straight men in football shirts substantially too tight for them to uphold any dignified masculinity. It was not the best setting for a queer awakening, although there was one drag queen singing most weeks called Kat-Sue Curry, who, given my close affinity with the dish, became a firm favourite of mine, and so the night had a touch of camp about it.

Each Thursday during my first term I would watch Nick get up to belt out a rendition of Take That's 'Shine' – week upon week upon week upon week. Whilst some humans get bored of the monotony of having one karaoke song, Nick absolutely lapped it up. I would cheat on my newfound love of white Zinfandel rose and get in a four-pint pitcher jug of Kronenberg and start downing it to try to impress him, adopting all the toxic elements of a 'straight acting' identity, which I thought would, in the long run, make him like me more, and which was a huge rookie error.

Most of the straight male mates in our extended uni friendship group had completely accepted his sexuality without question, so a lot of Nick's hang-up's about his sexuality mainly came from his own internalised anxieties and shame – something I could palpably relate to. As you've read in the beginning few pages of this book, I was always worried about my own presentation of masculinity, fearful, I guess, that I was gay. However, by the time I reached my latter teens and after all the trauma of losing Dad, I was finally ready to explore this possibility.

In the back of my mind, whilst all of my and Nick's straight mates in this first year were out having mad casual sex with girls, I'd dreamt up a scenario whereby me and Nick would get drunk, I'd tell him I was gay, he'd tell me it was all OK and then somehow we'd immediately start romping. And while, yes, I wouldn't have had a clue what to do in a 'romp', it wouldn't matter because Nick was the wise old age of twenty-one and Georgia said he'd 'been to Thailand a few times on cheap backpacking holidays and once fucked a lad in the jungle'.

However, this scenario I'd dreamt up was just a fantasy manifesting in my head that the first gay guy I came out to would suddenly fall madly in love with me. This only ever happens in pretty terrible coming out videos on YouTube. And, in retrospect, now in 2020, I can honestly tell you that my only 'type' is someone who has never googled 'Cheap flights to Thailand'. *That is my ONLY type.*

What did happen was that me and Nick became slightly better friends. One time I saw his halls bedroom and realised that he was so obsessed with football and had completely different interests to me, and I knew deep down that I'd never fit the bill of an alluring romantic companion. Despite this, I also knew that I still trusted him to be one of the first people I came out to.

Much of my first year of university was spent daydreaming, pondering and strategizing how I was going to tell my friends – the location, the tone of voice I'd use, the reaction I hoped to receive and what the worst-case scenario could be. It would all be plotted out and built up in my head and then, in the nervousness of the moment, I'd discard everything and mostly just blurt out 'I think I'm gay!'

This is pretty much what I did to Nick.

One night, after a party round his halls flat, I waited hours for everyone to leave. Eventually, once the last duffle-coated visual art student with a Morrissey tattoo had closed the kitchen door, it was just me and Nick.

'I think I might be bi, or gay. I don't really know.'

Nick said very nonchalantly, 'OK … well that's fine.'

I think he'd maybe clocked why I'd been hanging around so much. We spoke about my feelings towards guys, that I knew I was sexually attracted to them but had had too much on in my teens with losing Dad to even explore that part of me, and so none of my close friends or family knew any of these feelings. Then we spoke about his sexuality, the fact he came out to some friends at eighteen, yet four years later he was still not out to his family. He told me how they'd been subtly led to believe he might be seeing a girl at our uni, as she was in ALL his Facebook photos, and he hadn't told them otherwise.

Once I felt a sense of relief that I'd finally told him after weeks of waiting, he leaned over the kitchen table and sternly asked for my discretion about him being gay. I understood and I asked for that same promise of discretion. He said we could go to some gay bars together, he'd take me under his wing almost – but the deal was, don't speak about it to people other than those who already know.

Now, there's a valid protection in sharing the principle of discretion with someone. In knowing your secrets are safe with one another. But it also can sow an early seed of damage. Somewhere in your brain, discretion reminds you that you have a secret you have arranged to keep from the world at large. Obviously, I don't mean I need everyone on planet earth to know I'm gay – despite what some of my Twitter jokes might proclaim! But what I do need is to feel comfortable being gay out in the world and, unfortunately, early on in the realisation of my sexuality, I was already putting terms and conditions on ensuring its concealment.

As my first year of university continued, me and Nick began to speak more and more about gay stuff: Grindr, dating, porn, drugs, the tribes of gays on campus. He would educate me through his personal lens of being gay and therefore that started to become mine. And as our friendship grew, it became clearer that I was starting to fancy him.

I began to feel hurt watching him chatting up guys I knew that he fancied. Seeing him flirt with boys who possessed a far superior physique to mine felt like stabs to the stomach. Knowing Nick would be sat in the corner of house parties, scrawling though Grindr, seeking out fun that he could so easily procure. And I had foolishly pinned my whole trust, understanding and the status of my sexuality on him and whatever our relationship was. And that wasn't really fair on him, nor me. Our relationship was only ever going to be platonic.

Rather than accept this, I did the age old thing of trying to change myself to fit whatever he found attractive. So I started going down the gym. I stopped eating ALL carbs. Some days I didn't eat full stop. This hadn't even happened with the stress of my dad's death, yet now I was starving myself to impress a closeted gay lad from Crewe. I became increasingly obsessed with the idea I could lose buckets of weight, cut my hair short and model myself into Nick's ideal guy. And as I did this – lost half a stone, then a stone, slightly trimmed my hair, trimmed it even shorter, lost a stone and a half – I received all the compliments and positive reinforcement that come with visible weight loss.

I'd go home and everyone would say, 'Oh Jack, you look great!' An XL from Zara would actually fit me! Imagine that, me dressed in mainland Spain's most petite male clothing line! Even my brother Dean, who hadn't been in the slightest bit interested that I'd even got into university, told me 'well done' on the weight loss. But I hadn't done it for anyone else, not even me. I'd done it to impress Nick. And even after losing nearly two stone, I still felt consumed with sadness watching him flirt with any other guys.

I would stand outside his halls block and stare at his window, knowing he was in there with someone that wasn't me. This was not healthy behaviour, it was an infatuation that I didn't understand until I was fully heartbroken.

One night I'd had enough. Our whole group had gone out for a BYOB curry, a lethal combination of cheap booze and food so spicy that any of our uni mates from the West Country got the shits from just a poppadom and some lime pickle chutney. I got blind drunk on six or seven glasses of trusty Blossom Hill Zinfandel and dipped one plain naan into some yoghurt and mint sauce to limit my calorie intake. At the end of the night, stood outside the curry house, I drunkenly told Nick that I fancied him. That he was someone I wanted more than a friendship with.

He sighed with the inconvenience of my admission. In all fairness to him, he did the right thing, telling me to go back home and sleep off the booze and forget about it in the morning. But I told him I couldn't. I told him I felt like I was falling for him and everything had become too hard.

In the frustration of it all, he told me it was never going to happen. I left.

Georgia and Dom came to find me in my room that night, having clocked I was clearly upset. However, some other mates followed them in and everyone sat around my bedroom trying to figure out how the new phenomenon of e-cigarettes worked. All of the wider group knew that Nick was gay, though Georgia and Dom were the only two friends who knew I was 'bisexual' at this point. Some of the others started speaking about Nick, how he wasn't your typical 'out there' gay guy.

I remember one lad, a rugby type called Rhys, proclaiming to the group: 'It is kinda weird Nick's gay, 'cause he doesn't seem to have been brought up to be one.'

A few awkward glances were exchanged across the room.

My friend Dom said, 'But you're born gay. You're not brought up gay.'

And Rhys replied, 'Well I dunno about that, 'cause my mum reckons it's nurture not nature, right, 'cause she had this friend who had this son who is now gay, and she were always letting him hang out with girls and wear nail varnish and see that lesbian popstar in concert. Whassur name? The one who's always swinging about on the trapeze.'

Georgia replied, 'P!nk.'

Rhys nodded. Eyes rolled around the room. Dom managed to take the conversation away from the nature-nurture debate but I had just frozen, sat there in my own room, shrinking inside myself. I wasn't articulate enough at the time to say what I felt or defend what I believed, so all I did was joke it off.

'P!nk is not a lesbian! Most lesbians would be too cool to have an exclamation mark in their name,' I said, in a dead-pan tone suggesting I wanted everyone to leave.

As the group gave up on e-cigarettes and went outside for a real one, Georgia turned to me privately and asked if I was OK. I told her Nick had said he didn't want me. And she shrugged and said, 'It's probably for the best. He's probably a bit jealous of you anyway.'

In bewilderment I replied, 'How?'

Nick was the kind of guy who placed a heavy importance on success, prestige and looking the part. Like quite a few gay guys I've met subsequently, there is an impulse in some of them to compensate for an internalised shame with looking, externally, like a big success. To either present an image that's far away from 'queerness' or 'vulnerability' or to try to be defined by something other than what they may, deep down, feel is still a 'problematic' sexual preference. I felt that Nick thought his own sexuality, at times, to be unfortunate. It is not for me to judge this behaviour; it can be to some a form of protection and I think some gay men don't even realise they're doing it. When we were growing up in the nineties and noughties, there was still very little education on same-sex relationships. It's only in relatively recent British history that Thatcher's government enforced 'Section 28', whereby many LGBTQ+ individuals were brought up in a culture that bred so much internalised shame in closeted queer people and where the visibility, promotion and normalisation of same-sex relationships was restricted by law.

Nick could also be very competitive. In our first year of university I was doing rather well, getting high marks in class and already doing bits of professional work at radio stations. Whilst I wasn't sure what my sexuality was, I still had a strong sense of who I was and what I wanted to be – I think because losing Dad had made me more driven. I knew my strengths, weaknesses and, importantly, my character. Whereas Nick perhaps hadn't fully accepted himself yet, embroiled in many different contracts of 'discretion'. (Though I really, really don't want to sound mean about Nick, because we were all very young and, if anything, he was very kind to me.)

After that night at the curry house, some distance between us grew. We were still friendly, but not close. I needed to get over my feelings, and so I didn't go out seeking a new gay friend or putting pressure on myself to do so because I knew that I needed to accept my sexuality myself before I expected anyone else to. So I stuck with the bunch of pals I already had who were mostly straight but were more than supportive.

One night, after a day of helping out with the student union's charity week, Georgia and I decided to stay in when everyone else was going to Messi Mondayz. She very sweetly concocted a plan for just us, something to cheer me up. So, we sat in her halls kitchen and drank a whole bottle of white Zinfandel – each. And at around 10pm she revealed her master plan: for us to get on the last train into London so I could lose my gay club virginity.

I nervously agreed and, two hours later, we were walking through the streets of Soho. Georgia relished in the opportunity to go dancing in a club whilst wearing the shortest Topshop mini skirt you could ever hope to buy.

Now, it's quite scary going to your first gay club, because the vast majority are all called things like 'Savage' or 'Envy' or 'Revenge'. It doesn't matter where you are in Britain, you're sure to find a tacky gay boozer named after a deadly sin, screening back-to-back Madonna videos on sticky 32-inch TV screens. I'm not sure if these club names are intended to be empowering or mainly just to create a melodramatic vibe of bitchiness and excitement, but I just felt like, why not call your gay bar 'Nice To Each Other', or 'Be Less Vain', or 'Who cares if my T-shirt's from River Island, they actually do some quite good stuff'?

After failing to find anywhere I wasn't terrified of, Georgia decided we should hit up G-A-Y bar on Old Compton Street. She said, and I quote her verbatim, 'The drinks are £1.60 and no one's gonna try and finger me on the dance floor.'

As we ran down Old Compton Street in Soho, we went past all the iconic gay pubs that held so much history about a community I had no education of. I had never been taught or learnt about the Admiral Duncan bombing, nor did I know about the Stonewall riots in NYC that led to the global Pride movement. But in that moment it was just me and my mate Georgia, drunkenly holding hands and acting like those most innocent of eighteen-year-olds on a night out in the city, running around with no real clue what they're doing.

We arrived and G-A-Y was closed. The night was not going well. We got pounced on by about three of twenty identical twinky promo boys holding stacks of neon-coloured. We grabbed two of them, which gave us free entry to a mega gay club called Heaven. This was it! My first proper gay club.

Georgia and I lined up for two hours outside Heaven, making friends in the queue with flamboyant gay-night regulars and other fresh-out-the-closet uni students. This was peak Gaga era, so, as you can imagine, every five minutes someone would be playing a very tinny .mp3 of 'Born This Way' from a shit android phone. Once, at last, we'd finally reached the very front of the queue, we got rejected by security because Georgia ... had a *knife* in her bag! An actual knife, from a charity bake sale we'd done earlier in the day.

Despite having flyers for the bake sale in her bum bag to prove it, we were removed from the queue and that was it. We'd been in London for three hours, not drinking, not dancing and the only solace we could find was that Georgia was right that she wouldn't be non-consensually or consensually fingered.

Shivering with cold, the two of us got the N18 bus for the 73-minute long journey all the way back to Harrow with a share box of twenty McNuggets and, again, watched more *Gavin & Stacey* in bed. But the sentiment was there. I had been to the gay district, as a gay man, with a friend who was completely there for me – even if she was totally drunk, disorganised and concealing weapons about her person.

how to help a loved one accept their sexuality

1 Listen up.

It is so important to just be an open-minded, supportive listener when someone is trying to broach the topic of sexuality to you. Remember that they may have been painstakingly planning this chat with you, going over and over it in their minds for days, weeks, months, even years. This is them revealing something incredibly personal, so be sure to remain as focused on them as possible and respect what they are and aren't willing to share.

2 No sticking labels.

The worst thing about 'coming out' for me was a definitive label being placed on me that I didn't really understand too much at the time and was maybe quite scared of. There's definitely a difference between accepting your sexuality/sexual preferences and also accepting a linguistic description of your whole identity.

Nowadays, we're so lucky that more language is coming into popular usage to help describe someone in this process of acceptance to feel a sense of identity, such as 'questioning' or just overarching terms like 'queer'. I think, first and foremost, when someone has come out to you as 'not straight', so to speak, make sure you don't reply to them with rigid labels. Don't say, 'So you're gay then?', because they themselves might still not fully know and they don't need an imposition. Ask questions in return that are open ended and allow them to explain the nuances of how they feel they might identify.

3 Don't be smug.

There is nothing worse than someone saying, 'I always knew, I knew it, I knew it!' like your sexuality was some sort of blatant secret you were keeping, or like they'd predicted who was going to win *Strictly* after week one. Please don't do this, it's really not useful. Things take time and you've got to respect that. Someone may have lived a whole life knowing they didn't meet certain stereotypical 'gendered' criteria to the outside world, and so you reminding them of this at such a delicate time can make them feel quite shit. Just wait until they're perfectly comfortable with their sexuality before telling them kindly if you had any 'suspicion'. And please discourage anyone else from reacting like I've described above to someone in those initial conversations.

4 Don't make it about you.

What I mean by this is that, if someone comes out to you, don't apply that immediately to how it may affect your life. (Although one time I came out to a friend who immediately celebrated the fact, saying 'a gay wing-man is the best wing-man', and I was both annoyed but also chuffed with this reaction.)

When my friend Lewis came out to me as a vegan, I let myself down by shouting, 'WHY ARE YOU DOING THIS TO ME WHEN YOU ARE THE ONLY PERSON IN OUR HOMETOWN I KNOW WHO CAN DRIVE AND WHO ALWAYS TAKES ME FOR A MCDONALD'S DRIVE-THRU IN WATFORD WHEN I COME HOME FOR CHRISTMAS?!'

But then Lewis reminded me that he could still drive me to McDonald's even though he was a vegan and he also told me to get the fuck over myself and now I'm very proud of him and his numerous beetroot-salad-stained Tupperware boxes.

5 **Respect the spectrum.**
This is important. If you, like me, subscribe to the idea that sexuality is on a spectrum, then don't be shocked if someone changes their position on that spectrum. It is perfectly normal for someone's sexuality to change or adapt as they grow older or become more accepting of who they really are.

I came out as bisexual first before now identifying as gay. And yes, it's a bit of a cliché. Many gays wrongly like to think of bisexuality as a holding pen, a sort of green room before going into the studio audience live record of flagrant homosexuality, series one, episode one. For me at the time, though, bisexuality felt like a valid part of my sexuality. I fancied some girls. I still do fancy some girls. But I just know that I don't want to be in a relationship with one. Please be as supportive as possible if someone changes how they feel and what they believe their preferences to be.

6 Understand internalised homophobia.

This is a bit of a serious point and I think it's very important, given the previous chapter. We unfortunately have a history of a heteronormative dominant culture, in all aspects of our media, storytelling and culture. Whilst great strides have been made and still are being made to diversify this, people growing up who think they might be LGBTQ+ today can still feel this sense of normal *vs* non-normal.

Internalised homophobia is when you are conditioned to believe that queer sexual preferences are wrong or negative, even if you may have started to indulge in your own same-sex attraction impulses. It's very complicated and it isn't just experienced by closeted guys with wives and kids who go off secretly fucking rent boys, or any of the seedy mainstream portrayals in which 'internalised homophobia' is explored. It's something much more conditioned and dangerous and I have really had to tackle it in myself at numerous points in the last six or seven years. It can manifest itself in lots of different paranoias, self-doubts and abusive cycles of thinking about what one's sexuality means in the wider world. Please take some time to read up on it if you care about being a good ally to the LGBTQ+ community, because just because someone is ready to be open about their sexuality, it doesn't mean they realise just how conditioned they may have been to see themself as abnormal or undeserving of certain rights/ expectations that heterosexual people have.

Politically, at the time of writing, we are still only half a decade into same sex marriage being legalised. Most gay people who are currently between their late twenties and early forties grew up under Section 28, the legislation I previously mentioned, which was brought in by Thatcher to prohibit educating children about same-sex relationships/ attraction and to essentially bully LGBTQ+ people into feeling/becoming invisible from mainstream society. It's part of the reason why so many LGBTQ+ lives have been disproportionally lost to mental health issues and suicide, because of tactics to isolate and divide public opinion about non-heterosexual people.

Thankfully, Section 28 didn't last for ever, but its legacy sowed many seeds of shame in so many LGBTQ+ people. I believe it's crucially important for people helping someone realising their sexuality to understand the complexities of that shame and for us all to try our best to defeat it with education, love and acceptance.

7 Be understanding of each individual.

Not every sexuality coming out story is the same, despite all popular films, TV shows and West End plays always having posters featuring two white, muscled guys, maybe slightly damp from rain or sweat, kissing with both passion and despair in their eyes. Sadly, we have a real dearth of diverse mainstream depictions of the LGBTQ+ experience and hopefully that is changing more and more.

I think it's important to remember that not every LGBTQ+ person has had the same upbringing or cultural/religious backgrounds. There are differences which will make self-acceptance and broader acceptance of an LGBTQ+ person really tricky and it's important to respect that.

There are many different support groups now for those from less accepting communities, so do some research and see if there's any way you can get some specific help and guidance.

8 Be excited for them.

Finally, I think it is also very important that, regardless of preference, you help someone to see that any realisation of their sexuality is a brilliant thing. It's going to make them happier and more fulfilled, if they can find a way to fully accept it.

It's going to be a huge weight off the shoulders for many even just to say it for the first time and you're bloody lucky if you're one of the first few people they open up to. That shows an immense amount of trust in you.

Whilst I wouldn't recommend just whisking your first queer pal off to the nearest drag queen night, you can definitely always support someone 'non-straight' by perhaps going with them to a sort of entry-level gay venue, club or pub. Now, I wouldn't recommend too many straights taking their gay mates into some places, because I suppose gay spaces are gay spaces for a reason – but most of them (the best ones) are also hyper inclusive and welcoming to anyone and everyone, regardless of sexual preference. On my twenty-first birthday, my straight pal Dom took me to G-A-Y late and he had the time of his life. He got hit on seven times, politely declined the requests and bought me endless £1.60 rum and cokes all night long. And that's how to be an ally!

shit poems

October 2011–June 2012

During those initial years after losing Dad, I would, on occasion, indulge myself in writing rather shit grief poetry. I'm of the belief that anyone bereaved should be lawfully allowed, perhaps even encouraged, to pen between one and ten ropey poems about loss as part and parcel of the grieving process. Rhyming 'died' with 'cried', 'dead' with 'bed', 'up in the sky' with 'why did you die'… lines dripping with melodrama, raw emotion and tedious metaphor that can all be forgiven due to circumstance.

I guess writing poetry or lyrics can often help someone's brain to process all the many thoughts and feelings that come with the upheaval of death, allowing you to articulate how you feel in a way that feels apt, cathartic and somehow translatable to others who may not be experiencing your loss. And yet, despite this defence, I really do have to hammer home to you that the initial grief poetry I wrote was very, very, very shit.

When I started my journalism degree, our lecturers warned us that the first year of work was very formulaically news-focused, and I wanted to keep up doing more creative writing, because it was always how I'd worked out emotional or complicated things in my head. Whilst doing journalistic projects at the Roundhouse in Camden, I found out they also had an in-house poetry course, where a bunch of writers aged eighteen to twenty-five would meet every Sunday for a year of writing workshops, culminating in that group performing the following summer as a poetry collective around many of the big festivals. So I signed up for the course that started around the time I began my first year at uni and got in with my very shit grief poetry.

These workshops spanned October 2011 to June 2012, a time just before brilliant performance poets like Kate Tempest and Hollie McNish massively blew up. Back then, not every TV advert for a bank or a razor was a spoken-word piece, said in a faux-Hackney, east London accent and filmed on a misty cobbled street. Performance poetry was just at a new dawn, helmed by an exciting set of poets who had emerged thanks to YouTube and didn't care so much about the page but created for the stage.

The teacher on the project was a poet/author called Steven Camden, who went by the name PolarBear. He was a collaborator and pal of another poet/rapper called Scroobius Pip, who, in 2011, I was a huge fan of. Pip would come in and do guest workshops that taught us the importance to your mental health of picking up a pen to figure stuff out. His hypothesis was, if your body needs a gym to keep physically fit, so does your mind. This was also just before the boom in mainstream mental health awareness.

The participant group for these sessions was quite a mixed bunch of ten to fifteen young writers, some of them English Literature students who were already writing flowery poetry and performing at literary salons. Some of them were tourists from Camden Market who I think had gone a bit astray and signed up for a LOL. And finally there were people like me, who wrote just because it helped them process stuff. After the first two months of the course, there were only six of us left and we all belonged to that final group.

Despite the fact that one sixth of us (me) was a boy, we collectively and colloquially named our collective The VC, or The Vagina Collective, which was an incredibly crap name for a supposedly talented bunch of innovative creative writers.

As our weekly sessions went on, I developed a huge affinity with these five girls. We were from all over the UK, had completely different back stories, families and past traumas, and yet we met up religiously each Sunday and shared our biggest and darkest secrets, turning them into poems or stories or, in my case, just funny lists that rhymed. I often used these sessions to work out how I was feeling about losing Dad. How I was, deep down, still consumed with an anger and feeling of abandonment because he wasn't here to finish off the job of being a parent. And so I voiced these feelings in poems, because that felt less scary in a way.

*

One week, I told the whole group all about Nick Mathieson and my crushes on men, which I didn't understand yet or know how to articulate. I had never said this to anyone outside of university and the whole group were completely non-judgmental, supportive and understanding. It was almost like the Roundhouse poetry collective was heavily subsidised group art therapy.

When it came to reading our poems, I fell in love with performing. After hating feeling like 'The Boy Whose Dad Died' and the weird awkwardness that came with, all of a sudden I was publicly speaking about grief and turning that awkwardness into audience laughter. My poems ranged from a story about the lasagnes that were dropped off on our doorstep to the farty bereavement counsellor. Suddenly I had a platform and the opportunity to put all these experiences into something that felt, in many ways, like closure and acceptance. And whilst I didn't really love going to many spoken word nights – most of the time I had no idea what people's poems about engulfing forests were about – I stayed for the one person who'd get up and perform something honest, funny and true to them. And through watching others, I realised so many more people had been through experiences which I'd otherwise locked away.

One of the other girls in my collective, Cecilia, confessed to me after our first public gig that her mum had also died quite rapidly of cancer when she was ten. She told me how it had massively affected her older brother, Leo, who was gay and struggling back in her home town of Brighton. She too understood that need to get away, and she was also spending her first year of university living in London, away from a place that felt shattered by loss. I can't explain how almost infectious that conversation was, how relieved I was that someone else was going through that pain and was trying to articulate it, too. It made me feel much less alone. And so, as the Roundhouse poetry collective (the VC), we started to plan a summer of gigs at music festivals all across the country. Vags on tour!

how to encourage creativity/community as catharsis

I am a huge advocate of getting someone to pick up a pen and try to work out difficult feelings. It went from being my coping mechanism as a teenager to now becoming part of my work and career. Here are some tips, i.e. what I tell mates to do when trying to practise some sort of creativity as a cathartic outlet.

1 **Sit down and write absolutely anything.**
It could be on a blank sheet of paper, in your iPhone notes or on the back of a Boots receipt. Just list stuff or just start free-writing, jotting down anything that comes to mind. It can be as real or as abstract as you want it to be – just letting yourself have the time to stream out your thoughts can be incredibly valuable. It's how I've often written about grief, because that emotional experience can sometimes feel so locked inside, so difficult to get out and articulate. Sometimes it feels much easier to spew out those feelings than try to craft something that feels poignant and helpful.

2 If it looks right for you or someone you know, do explore alternative therapy methods such as art, music and drama therapy.

I myself have never done any of these in an official sense, but in many ways the poetry collective project felt like creative writing therapy. Each week was like a huge lifting from my shoulders of pent-up stories I wanted to share and get out of me. I have occasionally been sceptical over the years, seeing leaflets for very expensive art therapy courses, as I believe that a wide range of creative or artistic hobbies can be as inexpensive as a pen and paper or some cheap paint and brushes. Something that can really help people to feel calm, rooted and focused on creating something can be as symbolic of your emotions as you want it to be. Also, if someone has the money, then fuck it – try every bloody art therapy you can and tweet me which ones were great or shite.

3 Sign up to group activities.

I really recommend this, especially if you feel someone may have been quite isolated recently and could do with a challenge, but still with the safety of knowing others are in a similar boat. I'd recommend arts and crafts meet-ups, local choirs, book groups, writing groups like my poetry collective – anything where you'll be able to creatively focus whilst meeting new people can be really good for your mental health. Obviously, exercise-focused groups too, like meditation, yoga, gym, dance classes and any specific sports groups, can also be good for benefitting from that communal feeling.

Recently I discovered a new initiative called 'The Grief Network', which has been set up in London and has fast become incredibly popular. It's a semi-regular meet-up for young people to discuss grief in pubs and cafés, mixed with the odd creative workshop and some performances and talks relating to loss. Do some research and see if there is anything similar in your local area that could be about any issue which you or a friend has been affected by.

Sadly, we are living in an era of so many closures of our community centres, spaces, venues, pubs, clubs and libraries – all to make space for more commercial ventures and privately built blocks of flats. So I think it's now become more important to just regain as much communal activity as possible in our daily lives. I cannot hammer home enough the sheer solace I found in discovering other people who could also relate to what I was going through, who weren't already in my friendship group. This all came through engaging in creative projects. And, actually, when I feel most happiest as a human being (sorry to go all DEEP on you all), is when I've found common ground with a stranger, whether that is having both lost parents or coming out as gay or even just liking ITV daytime's programming schedule a bit too much. There is no better feeling for your mental wellbeing than connecting with someone you otherwise didn't know, so do some research and try something new.

condoms and calmzines

The first job I got at eighteen was predominately giving out free condoms to fellow students as the University of Westminster Harrow Campus Student Union and Welfare Services peer-student receptionist and administrator *exhale breath*.

Originally I got this job because I had to do 40 hours of student union volunteering each year as part of my scholarship and then, after that, I just stayed working on the reception in a paid role, partly because I enjoyed it but predominantly because the only other job interview I got was at Sports Direct in Harrow and they refused to give me a retail position due to 'a lack of sports knowledge'. (I had failed to identify Lionel Messi on a FIFA World Cup 2010 poster, but I was very adamant that 'I *do* know who Clare Balding is.')

The SU receptionist role involved three main tasks. Firstly, I had to give out NUS membership cards to those who cared very little that they were signing up to the longest running confederation of student unions in the United Kingdom, and just wanted 10 per cent off in Topshop.

Secondly, I had to give worried students the GUM clinic opening hours in the local area. And finally, I created a 'safe space' where essentially very horny students would feel comfortable procuring free contraceptives, *sans* judgement.

My condoms (I changed the pronoun to 'my', as frankly they were the only company I had in a tiny office) came in three sizes: Pasante Regular™, Pasante Big™ and Pasante King Size™ – all easily retrievable from three stainless steel buckets kept on the counter of the reception desk.

You could take away as many as you wanted, within reason, in a white-and-pink striped paper bag designed to provide the sexually active with a clever decoy so the condoms looked like your everyday bag of pick 'n' mix. This was, however, futile, as the pick 'n' mix sweet bags in the student shop were just brown, so everyone knew you were packing some johnnies – you dirty slut!

My condoms were very popular because they were situated in a barely frequented office, between our halls of residence and the Undercroft student bar, aka the student sex market.

However, this job came with a weird side effect.

It meant that very quickly I knew roughly how big everyone's penises were.

Including my friends' penises.

And this meant that very quickly I became the most powerful person on campus.

This was a power I never asked for but nonetheless one I possessed with kind discretion, like Spiderman's ability to anonymously rescue NYC or Mel C's ability to carry the whole band vocally but still split the royalties.

I was very respectful of confidentiality. However, I worked out that my mate Tom Bowens had a King Size™ dick. Additionally, I worked out my friend Ben[1] had a Regular™ dick. I won't use the word small because size doesn't matter, however Ben had a tendency to put his hands deep into the regular condom bucket, feeling each packet with his index finger and thumb to find the smallest ones. He was, in fact, rather open about it.

In the name of transparency, I'll say that I myself have been known to wear the regular size, a fact about which I possess no shame, though I have been told by some ex-fat lads that losing two stone or more means you can gain a half-inch or two. I'm far more concerned right now in gains being made by the far right in Europe than any potential phallic growth.

Then, one day, a guy came into the student union office with a very different dilemma. His name was 'Anonymous Name to Protect Identity' and he was a really sweet, very skinny and pretty attractive lad who sadly possessed all the confidence of Neville Longbottom in the first film, before he

---

[1]   This name has been changed to protect the privacy and dignity of this student. I should have done this with Tom's name but he probably loves the fact everyone knows he has a huge cock. Well done, Tom!

got really fit. (Have you seen photos of the actor Matthew Lewis now? My lord!)

Anyway, 'Anonymous' came in and said, trying to conceal embarrassment: 'Erm, I was just wondering if you had, any, bigger?'

Now, I did not believe this to be a boast. I believed this was a young man at the very end of his student maintenance grant eating predominantly super noodles with Lidl's low-salt soy sauce who needed free johnnies.

After a quick call to the local sexual health supplier, I discovered the wonderful world of ... Pasante Super King™! These condoms were so big I could fit three of my fingers in one and, I mean, my fingers are so fat, I have trouble sending a text! Sometimes I actually have to sit down to type, like my nan, if I want to achieve any accuracy in spelling – that's how fat they are!

The people at the condom company kindly sent a box of 12 Super Kings™ on a monthly basis to our SU, which I kept hidden for my special big boy, whilst also using the spare ones to double-up as incredibly effective water balloons during the summer months.

One day, Anne, the head of student welfare, called me into her office for a chat. She was in her late fifties, had short spiky red hair, rode a Kawasaki scooter and went on biking holidays with her fella. Her office was like a museum of the recent past, as it was adorned in 1990/2000s band posters, weird plastic troll dolls hanging off the walls and a map of the world with cocktail-stick flags in countries where students came from. She had basically created an environment where anyone from shy international first-years to paranoid stoner art-school kids could come, feel safe and talk to her without judgement. And she spoke so generously and frankly about having a full mental breakdown a few years before that you couldn't help but open up to her.

On this particular morning, Anne told me that we needed to display a new men's magazine next to the condom buckets.

'Are we encouraging male students to have posh wanks?' I joked to Anne.

She didn't know what a posh wank was, but she still laughed. Anne went on to say that it was a different sort of magazine. She was the first person to tell me that suicide was the single biggest killer of young men. She was starting to hear of more and more students and recent male graduates who'd taken their own life, either at university or shortly after leaving or dropping out. It was a waste of young life that Anne felt compelled to try to tackle.

She'd started talking to a charity called CALM – the Campaign Against Living Miserably – about how they could have a presence at our university and she handed me a stack of free magazines she wanted me stock next to the condoms, called the *CALMzine*. This was a free monthly culture, lifestyle and advice magazine aimed at young men, about young men and written by mostly young men, talking about everything from anxiety to dating to OCD to which drugs you should avoid if you don't want to shit yourself. It was brilliantly illustrated by some great artists and perfectly pocket-sized.

The advice features ran alongside entertaining interviews with emerging, hyped-up bands and cultural figures, who were on the front cover, all being asked not just about their work or new single, but most importantly about what they did to help their own mental health. This was back in 2012, before these sorts of conversations were a big part of our current media landscape.

I remember reading through and falling in love with it. It was mental health propaganda, but compiled in an accessible, funny, tongue-in-cheek and important way. It felt like something that genuinely would help those who needed it. CALM would use the zine to also raise awareness of their free suicide prevention helpline.

Anne knew that I'd love it, and after all I'd been through, it resonated with me so much, so we put piles of magazines next to each steel bucket of condoms and we soon ran out. The more I read them, the more I wanted to contribute, so I contacted CALM to see if I could write about what they were doing for my final year university project, which was to make a short-form media piece about an issue affecting our generation. They were totally up for it – anything that could get the word out about the charity amongst the student body.

I decided I wanted to make something about CALM to play on our student radio station, so I organised to meet up with the head of news, Olly, to discuss it.

meeting Olly

early 2012

On the surface, Olly was a Jack-the-lad type – good looking, well dressed and always holding a Red Stripe in every student night nightclub photo. When I met him he was twenty-four, a second-year journalism student who had a good five years on everyone else in his year and mine. His Twitter feed was a mix of funny gobshite opinions and jokes about politics, TV and Newcastle United – sports quips that mostly went right over my head. When I saw him at uni, he was always surrounded by a similarly good-looking bunch of second-year boys who I found intimidatingly fit.

This particular chat – about CALM and my final year project – would be the first time we'd spoken properly. We got on OK, but there was never any blossoming of friendship. To him, I was probably just the weird, overly keen fat lad with curly hair, and I don't think he really wanted to have this pint I'd asked him for.

After basic pleasantries and two pints of £1.90 lager in the SU bar, I soon brought up CALM and how I wanted to make a radio package about their suicide prevention campaign and magazine for the station. Olly straight away loved the idea, wanting to know more as he flicked through the zine, buzzing about it like I had. He very sweetly and openly told me he'd dealt with some of his own mental health issues and so the cause fully resonated with him and he'd support anything CALM and I were trying to do.

I was really surprised by his openness and told him a sort of truncated story about losing my dad and my last few years of grief. In return, Olly gave me his headlines: parents splitting when he was young, dad now living in Japan with a new family, him having tough teenage years and being very close with his nan and grandad. I think we both got the sense that, unlike some of our peers, we'd both had much tougher teenage years. This all came from chatting about CALM, which is often the beauty of a charity like that – a conversation-starter enabling people to open up about their own experiences.

Olly never went into too much detail about his mental health issues early on in our friendship, but I'd like to think this chat sowed a seed in his mind and made him aware he could talk about it. Depression or mental illness didn't faze me, even then. Whilst grief isn't necessarily a mental illness, some of the symptoms and long-lasting effects of a tragic loss can cause depression. And I had been very depressed, having spent days in bed unable to get past huge sadness. I understood it.

Then, out of the blue, Olly remarked, 'I've heard from people in your year that you, like, do poetry? Spoken word stuff?'

I told Olly that I'd started performing and was writing some poems, but that I thought most spoken word was a bit shit. He nodded in agreement, before confessing that he too wrote his own poetry. His tone of voice slightly changed and he spoke really passionately about how he loved a lot of hip hop lyricists, beat poets and newer spoken word acts like Scroobius Pip. I told Olly that I'd met Pip on my poetry course and that was it – a second round of drinks was bought, we were chatting poems.

Olly asked me to read some in the smoking area, and so I gave him a personal performance and he was chuckling, giving me silly solo rounds of applause and telling me what specific lines to tighten up or words to remove to improve my delivery.

'These aren't really poems, are they mate? They're just funny lists.'

We then aired our grievances about the spoken word 'voice', which I loathed – a sort of formulaic mimicry whereby performers would adopt an accent different to their speaking voice and place emphasis on random words, pausing within rhythms in ways that felt desperate or disingenuous or trying to feign poignancy. How so much was just kids trying to imitate performers like Kate Tempest.

Once we'd got a third round in, we back and forthed about our favourite lyricists and bands. I brought up my obsession with the rapper M.I.A, and he said he'd send me an email listing some 'proper rap', which I took offence to. (I'd eventually open this email, in which he listed about twenty nineties hip hop albums I must listen to, in 2017, following a random search of 'Wu Tang Clan' in my inbox.)

Olly said he had a tattoo of his favourite Stone Roses track 'I Wanna Be Adored' and I ribbed him for the arrogance of that, suggesting maybe that his interpretation was more that he wanted to be loved than adored, after which he told me to: 'Shut up mate, I just got it 'cause it's a bloody great song!'

I showed him the design of a paper plane that I wanted tattooed on my top arm in tribute to M.I.A, a design I have showed many people thousands of times for the best part of the last decade, despite still not actually having a single tattoo to date.

The fourth round of drinks was bought, and by now Olly and I were properly drunk, loudly ranting on about life. About how so many art-school kids at our university could be so blindly privileged. And how we were the first in our families to go to university and didn't feel like those back at home fully understood what we wanted to do. And then we spoke about how we'd both been on waiting lists to see counsellors when we felt like shit. For the first time I could see his vulnerability.

I got the fifth round in, noticing Olly drunkenly open up even more. His accent, his tone of voice, could almost be quite goofy at times, with a southern twang reminiscent of mine. His voice would chuckle and quiver when he spoke passionately. It was honest, frank, considered. He wasn't overly verbose or anything, but he said things to you in a certain rhythm, like he'd lived a life of 100 years and had come back in time to tell me about what he'd learnt. He was a jumble of character traits: confident yet shy, sweetly silly yet severe in his reckonings on the world. He didn't match up to any of my preconceptions about him and so I felt a huge sense of comfort in speaking to him. To someone who came from a similar world to me.

Olly told me he'd gone to an all-boys state school in Chichester that was a bit rough and had grown up immersed in masculinity. And I could still sense this bravado about him, to the point where I felt like I didn't want to refer at all to my sexuality because, in the back of my mind, I wasn't sure if he had any gay friends, or whether he was really that 'cool' with the gays. This was very much a symptom of my own paranoia.

Olly told me he worked at Sainsbury's for a while after he finished school. He never thought he'd make it to university because he didn't have the qualifications, but his then girlfriend, who was planning to go to uni in London, helped motivate him on to an access course to get the qualifications so that he could apply. He knew he wanted to study to become a journalist. Our university didn't initially give him a place, so apparently he called the course leader and, with the gift of the gab, blagged his way in. It was his one last chance at higher education. Considering all he'd done to get there, it was such an amazing story of persistence and I was so inspired by that. That determination to invest in himself.

The sixth round of drinks came with some disgusting cherry Sourz shots as a crap third-year DJ clambered on to the SU decks, playing bad dubstep for a few hours, which we drunkenly danced to before calling it a night.

Outside the bar we swapped numbers and he hugged me, coyly remarking, 'I'd really like, if you were up for it, for you to read some of my poetry sometime?'

'Of course,' I replied. 'Why don't I come round yours in the summer for a writing day?'

'I don't live round here, unfortunately, I live in Willesden,' Olly said, with the same disgruntled tone that any student who *lived in Willesden* would have used to proclaim that. Willesden wasn't too far from Harrow, but it wasn't a glamorous place you necessarily ever wanted to go unless you were getting the bus to IKEA.

There was something about Olly where I felt like, in this one night, we'd kind of agreed we wanted to spur each other on to succeed. This is something I've often found with other working-class kids aspiring to get somewhere, that we kept an eye out, wanting to root for each other in turning our adversity into determination and, ultimately, happiness.

I told him, 'Well, I can travel to Willesden or you could come perform at a poetry open mic with me sometime?'

Olly smiled. He'd never read any of his poems aloud to a room full of people but agreed to just read some to me first.

'I write all my poems on my phone notes and I'm not really a performer. And I'm not really competitive,' he said.

'Open mics don't have to be a competition. I'm not really into doing wanky poetry slams,' I replied, naively.

He nodded and we agreed to meet after the summer. And that night was the beginning of one of the most important friendships I've ever had.

the Olympically gay summer of 2012 – part one

Summer 2012

In June, I finished my first year and moved out of halls, kissing goodbye to Karen in the accommodation office and the need to lie about having restless legs syndrome.

At the end of BA Multimedia Journalism Year 1, the scores were:

Guys Fucked – 0

Dicks Sucked – 0

I should say at this point that I did try to explore heterosexuality in my first year one night, by engaging in a sexual act with a girl called Gemma. It was doomed from the off and lasted about 25 seconds. Gemma is now someone who I'm still friends with (mainly interacting via mutual likes on Facebook) and, despite what some of my mates would say, I did NOT get with Gemma just because she got 15 per cent off in Bella Italia! (Although, sadly, this didn't include the Leicester Square branch, as I had to find out the hard way!)

I also had my first same-sex kiss in that year. It was with a boy called Louis under a tree in the fields beside our campus, where around thirty of us were dangerously undercooking meat on cheap disposable barbecues. Louis and I kissed about three times and then Louis left without saying goodbye. I was devastated. When I departed the undercooked barbecue tree, I saw Louis kissing another boy under another tree. I had been tree-cheated on. One could call it tree-ason.

Just like uni students everywhere, once I was out of halls I was back at home spending the summer at my childhood house. This meant lying in my bedroom and pretending to be straight again. Though going on Grindr back in my hometown was always exciting, because one by one I could see who from my primary school was also turning out gay and who from secondary school ended up loving the D! (Ironically, it's usually the boy who called you a fag for coming last in cross country who's now desperately sending pictures in a knitted jockstrap!)

But that summer, amongst the buzz of the London 2012 Olympics, I thought about telling my mum the truth about the feelings I was having. The fact that all five of the Spice Girls had reunited and performed at the opening ceremony standing on the roofs of London black cabs felt like a sign from Dad. That he'd made the Spice Girls reunite in the campest spectacle ever seen in international sports and wanted me to come out as a big ol' gay.

However, every time I thought about 'coming out', I remembered when Todd kissed Nick on *Coronation Street* – an iconic first for early noughties television. I watched it with my mum, feeling weirdly intrigued by it all, and then I saw her quite casually wince and then remark, 'Uhhh, I wish they wouldn't put it right in your face!'

Now, my mum would wince any time she saw any sex or kissing scene on TV, but there was something about that comment that stuck with me. Whilst I knew she wasn't an out-and-out homophobe, I do feel that my mum, like many other parents her age, was very conditioned in a heteronormative culture. And I guess I felt like she'd just really worry about me if she knew I was gay.

Around this time I thought I might tell my eldest brother, Al, but then I remembered one day in Year 11 when he took me shopping for school shoes. I'd picked out and tried on a pair of skinny pointed brogues in New Look, but Al wouldn't buy me them because he said they looked 'gay!' (The irony being that nowadays I often see Al wearing a pair of pointed brogues!)

Telling my middle brother, Dean, about any homosexual thoughts I was having never even crossed my mind, and so, ultimately, I kept my feelings about my sexuality to myself. Never once did I think my family would ever ridicule me, or cast me out or love me less, but I did feel that, deep down, they just wouldn't want me to be gay. And so they wouldn't feel able to be happy for me. This completely wasn't true, but, back then, I made these little promises to myself to keep schtum. I'd carry on being privately, 'discreetly' gay but make sure I didn't engage in anything too public, so no one back home would catch wind. And anyway, aside from kissing some lad by a tree, I hadn't actually done anything that remotely denoted gay behaviour. I hadn't even successfully gained entry into a gay club, and they let just about any old fucker in!

This summer was also about doing lots of gigs with the poetry collective, and suddenly, despite slagging off poetry slams to Olly, I had found myself non-consensually signed up to perform in one! The collective had been booked to kick off our summer gigs at a festival called Meadowlands, a tiny little boutique arts weekender in a field near Brighton with around 2,000 punters. None of us actually read the initial email stating that the gig would take the form of a poetry slam because we'd all been too excited at the prospect of getting pissed up and being paid £25 along with a free burrito voucher. Then, whilst checking my emails one afternoon, I read some correspondence from a festival organiser saying that I needed to prepare 'a two-minute slam piece to read in front of a midnight audience of potentially very pissed, very high festival goers'. It was my worst nightmare.

But then, two weeks before the slam, something terrible happened. Whilst at a warm-up gig, Cecilia from our collective found out that her brother Leo had taken his own life. He was only nineteen. We'd all only known Cee for the best part of nine months, and yet spending every Sunday with her, and performing together, made her feel like family. I was utterly devastated for her. So many of Cecilia's poems were in some way about loss: losing her mum aged ten, re-building her life afterwards in Brighton and eventually finding teenage love as an escape from it all – her words felt tinged with sadness mixed with an undefeatable hope.

Leo's death was the first time I had indirectly known of a young male taking his own life, and it was the first time that I saw just how strong a sense of character Cecilia has.

We told Cecilia that she could do whatever she wanted about the summer of gigs we'd booked ahead but, as was her nature, she Trainlined the fuck out of group rail tickets, stole a pop-up tent off a lad she was shagging and off we all went – me, Cee, and two more poets, Jess and Maria – to do exactly what we'd planned: get shitfaced together in a field near Brighton. Cecilia wanted to regain some normality after losing Leo, to get back on the wagon of performing again and, I guess, to not let tragedy win. I was in awe of her.

We arrived at the festival, threw up two pop-ups in the artist campsite and opened a bottle of wine, each. Naturally mine was a £5 Blossom Hill white Zinfandel. (This was very much the final days of my Zinfandel obsession, before we ended our relationship, and nowadays I can't even smell a glass of rosé without feeling mildly nauseous.)

The poetry slam took place in a tiny bell tent, cramming in approximately sixty to seventy drunk revellers. They were bohemian, arty Brighton types – not the sorts you'd see nowadays in Lucy & Yak dungarees with arts administrator jobs, but really fusty, hippy, organic types. Men and women wearing hemp hoodies and sporting matted dreadlocks passed round spliffs, despite all being very, very white. It was a bit dodgy.

By midnight I was pissed and incredibly nervous as I went to perform one of my sad grief poems. The piece I'd prepared for the gig was dreadful. I mean D-R-E-A-D-F-U-L.

And thus, my first slam performance went a little like this:

'Hi, I'm Jack, is this on? Yep? Great. I'm from Watford, I'm in my first year of uni and I'm a part of the Roundhouse Poetry Collective and this poem is called – what sorry? Yes, OK, yes, I'll get on with it! Sorry for the preamble. This poem is called "Character Building".'

[Pre-performance cough, sip of warm Strongbow, deep breath.]

When I was 14 the McCanns lost their Maddie.
When I was 15 cancer took away my daddy and,
When I was 16 everybody was a baddy –
'Cause what I'd lost could never now be found.

Yes. That was an actual first verse of a poem I performed in front of other human beings, comparing my dad's untimely death to that of international child abduction! Brace yourselves for more, thankfully less diabolic prose ...

And now when I stand,
I stand with one foot on the ground
The other in the grave;
Of a childhood paved
With empty ending spaces.
Some call me brave,
'Cause that's how they compute it –
Sugar coat it
Water it down
Then just totally dilute it,
With phrases like –
'I know how it feels.'
As if a warm friendly connection
With a mate, neighbour or stranger
is gonna erupt through dad dying
and 'you' sharing that experience,
Sharing 'it'.
I understand that phrase is a mechanism people pull out,
When they have little else to say but,
It is always you who must smile
to tell everyone
'It's Character Building!
 It's actually totally built me as a person, like, I don't even
            need to go on a gap yah to Africa anymore!'
But actually,
it,

grief,
it renders your character temporarily fucked.
'No building today!
Just sitting down
With a stay at home mum
Being a stay at home son
Watching Loose Women.
On a bed of losing lottery tickets
A mountain of unwashed mugs
And a stack of month old tv guides!'
That's not character building –
That's bereavement.

But I suppose the long term effects of the latter do matter
And grief has changed me as a person.
But whether or not it has built me
Is something I am yet to find out.

I know this is not the best piece of verse, but I do think there is something quite sweet about this shit poem, about eighteen-year-old me trying to make sense of everything I'd gone through. Because, at twenty-five, I can now look back and say that bereavement *has* actually built my character, but back then it felt more like it had destroyed it.

And besides, somehow I won the slam. Out of twelve poets, I was crowned Meadowlands Festival 2012 Spoken-Word Slam Winner and I'm still as shocked as you are.

The judge of the slam was picked out randomly from the audience. He was some bloke from Bristol who, on awarding my victory, said to the crowd, 'Any fucker brave enough to do a Madeleine McCann joke gets my vote!' whilst clasping his hands around my shoulders, like I was his son who'd scored the winning goal at a football match.

I said, 'That wasn't a Madeleine McCann joke.'

And he said, 'Well, it made me laugh!'

I was mortified. Bristol bloke was so high he then fell over on to a decorative cactus, such was the level of artistic merit held by the audience at this poetry slam.

I collected my trophy from the organisers of the event, who turned out to be a really fun bunch of stand-up poets in a collective called Bang Said the Gun. They liked my 'gap yah' joke and said that I should carry on writing funnier stuff, and they invited me to come down to their open mic night in London. I agreed to do it after the summer.

After the slam everyone continued getting pissed until, one by one, the stragglers drifted off drunkenly to their tents, leaving just me and Cecilia sat outside a 'Mexican' food stall run by a couple from Crawley. I asked Cee how she was doing and she smiled, took both of my hands and said, 'Shall we get some chicken nachos, yeah?'

So, surrounded by fumes of spliffs and flares, we sat eating quite possibly the saddest bowl of chicken-coated microwaved nachos I'd ever had. Our chat soon drifted to Leo, and Cecilia told me more about his troubles, how she had tried so many times to save him as a teenager – rescuing him from self-sabotage, harm and substances that were never going to help. I told her it's no one's responsibility to save someone, that all you can do is love them, and she nodded, wiping a tear from her face. She said she wished somebody would save her sometimes. I felt the same.

We sat hand in hand on the bench, our elbows unavoidably drenched in other people's sour cream and guacamole from the day, and Cecilia told me that, because Leo was so confused about being gay, it was another part of himself he had struggled to accept in many ways. There was something in the safety of mine and Cecilia's chat that made me feel I could tell her anything, and so I said that I thought I was gay. That I wasn't really 'bisexual'. And thus, in that moment, I almost left the purgatory of whatever that label meant to me.

Back then, I believed that bisexual people could just easily assimilate into the optics of mainstream 'heterosexual' relationships without causing much fuss and would be able to pop out children the old-fashioned way. Nowadays I know that this isn't strictly true, and that bisexual people still have their own stigmas to contend with. However, me gradually picking apart my conditioned mythological ideas that I had about different LGBTQ+ people was a huge part of figuring out my sexuality. I realised that most of those stereotypes that I believed in, about all different kinds of minorities, needed to just be chucked in the bin. That they were born out of a prejudice that I didn't myself harbour but that culture and a lack of education in these groups had conditioned in me.

Pulling out two cans of lager that we'd stolen from backstage, Cecilia told me to never be ashamed of whatever I was. That my mum, brothers and everyone would and *should* love me regardless, just like she loved Leo.

In that moment, I showed her that I had Grindr on my phone. Even though I'd still never used it, we sat chuckling and scrolling from the tops to the bottoms, Cecilia's mind blown by the proximity of men who were willing to send anonymous, introductory dick pics. She made me promise not to take on any shame about this stuff, that it was a valid part of me that I needed to explore, and with this final gift of wisdom we drifted off back to our tents, arm in arm, clasping near-empty cans of Heineken.

I flopped into my tent at around 2am and realised that, for the first time as an adult, I was fully on my own and away from home. Not just 15 minutes down the road at uni, but in a totally new environment where I was completely anonymous. No one here knew who the hell I was, apart from my fellow poets, one Bristolian man with a terrible sense of humour and about sixty other stoned spoken-word fans. So, I decided to hit up Grindr and see if there was anyone in the surrounding fields who was gay. I'm not sure what my intentions really were, as I lay there on an inflatable lilo on a warm summer's night, but soon enough a message flashed up from a guy called Pete.

We initiated what I now know to be some fairly classic hook-up messaging – the back and forth, the obvious formulaic pleasantries that come with a Grindr exchange's wheels in motion.

'Hey how're u?'

'Yh good thanks. How're u?'

'Yh good thanks. What u up to?'

'Horny?'

'Same.'

'Where r u??'

This script is nowadays just as much a part of gay male culture as Judy Garland in *The Wizard of Oz*.

Soon enough, I was traipsing through three different fields with another horrible can of Strongbow in hand (dark fruits, I'm not a monster), looking around and trying to find Pete's tent.

As I entered what I hoped was Pete's campsite, I scoured the litter of mismatched tents. All I knew from his Grindr messages was that his tent was roughly underneath a flag that read 'TONY BLAIR'S A MURDERER'. Intense.

I was drunk, nervous, shy, yet desperate for just anything to happen. For any intimacy to manifest itself in any way. I wasn't necessarily after tent shagging, but I guess I just wanted to relinquish myself over to something, something that had always felt so in-built and inevitable, and to see what happened.

I found the Blair flag and walked towards Pete, who was waving and smiling, looking slightly worse for wear. He was thirty-two, had a septum piercing and had eyes like the demon headmaster – all things I thought I was totally into. His profile said he was an employee of the natural body product brand LUSH and Pete seemed perfectly nice, but it was soon evident that he definitely just wanted a tent shag and that I was far too nervous.

We started chatting and he told me he was at the festival with his job and this was enough for me to trust that he must be a fairly good guy. My theory was that, if you work for LUSH and you think Blair's a war criminal, you're probably a bit angsty but a sweetheart nonetheless. So, awkwardly, Pete and I tried to clamber into his tent. However, I immediately noticed someone else was also in there, asleep.

'Ah, that's my mate, Darren. He's taken so much ketamine he thinks he's at Butlins right now,' quipped Pete.

After accidentally treading on 'Daz', we quickly aborted the tent plan. Pete suggested he could come to mine, but I was in artist camping, and fuck boys like him weren't allowed into the compound without an artist wristband, in case, I dunno, they tried to bundle on top of Dick and Dom or pinch a joint off Speech Debelle. (These were the two headline acts of the festival.)

So, instead, Pete and I just walked and walked and walked, through another three campsites or so, until we reached the only place deserted enough at 3.18am to engage in sexual activity without being caught … The Children's Field.

This Children's Field was open from 12 noon till 3pm for parents to take bohemian little Bellas and Hugos for immersive theatre shows – otherwise known as watching some twenty-three-year-old drama school graduates shame themselves. But at 3am that night it was just me and Pete, sat alone on a bright yellow dandelion bench and Pete got his dick out. (It was very much our own theatre of shame.)

If you'd prefer to be spared the 'sheer erotica' of this next story, you may skip ahead a couple paragraphs, but if you're feeling brave then grab a Kinder Bueno and strap in!

Pete shoved my face on his willy and it was disgusting, because his dick tasted like the actual smell of a LUSH shop – that wall of synthetic sickly bubble-gummy stench which hits you every time you even walk slightly close to a LUSH branch. That was what my mouth was playing host to. It was the first time I had ever committed an act of fellatio and it felt like sucking off a foreskinned bath bomb.

So I took my mouth away from his genitalia and up to his lips so that we could kiss and even his mouth tasted like LUSH. It was all too much. Quickly he then pushed my head back down to his heavily perfumed penis, but as I went down slowly I suddenly heard Pete piercingly scream out.

'Ahhhhh for fuuuccckkkksss sakkkeeeeee!!'

I stopped.

I looked up.

A drop of blood fell on my T-shirt.

One of my curls had got tangled in Pete's septum piercing, and the further I was going down south, the more I was gradually mutilating his nostrils. In a panic, Pete violently ripped a clump of my curly hair out and we proceeded to find the nearest urgent medical assistance at the St John's Ambulance first aid tent. Saint John is actually the patron saint of saving drunk gays!

(Fun Fact: four years later, me and Pete matched on Tinder. He still works at LUSH but, sadly, no longer identifies as a member of the pierced septum community. His nose looked fine, though. I think.)

That next morning, I woke up and left Meadowlands festival with my poetry slam trophy poking out my backpack and the scream of Pete's injury still ringing in my ears.

Our next gig was the week of my nineteenth birthday, at the end of July 2012. I spent the night of my birthday on an overnight Megabus going up to the Edinburgh Fringe Festival. One member of our collective, Paloma, thought she'd take a sleeping pill to help her get through the ten-hour journey; however, she accidentally took the wrong pill, one with a certain high attached to it and she was pretty much buzzing off her tits from Milton Keynes to Carlisle.

Our poetry collective had a five-show run on the Free Fringe, an independent branch of the Edinburgh Fringe Festival, which runs alongside the main events. As you can probably tell by the name, entry to each show costs zero pounds and, in theory at least, audience members pay what they think it's worth at the end. There's limited financial risk performing on the free fringe, but performers still get to benefit from being amongst all the buzz and footfall of the world's largest arts festival. Our venue was a pub half an hour's walk from the festival hub, in the basement of a now closed-down establishment called the Fiddler's Elbow, in a room that sat around thirty-five people at a push.

The first performance ended in a rapturous closing applause from about six audience members, who generously donated a grand total of £13, or £2.30 each. We were 12 per cent of the way there to paying off our Megabus fare!

Our collection dipped down to £6 for our second show, then shot up to £23 the next day, then £47 the day after that, until finishing our run on the dizzy heights of £62.14! What a rags-to-riches story! Despite the lack of profit, we broke even on travel and we all had an absolute blast.

Once our five shows were over, I decided to stay for an extra week. I'd made friends with some performers who were on for the whole month, including two sketch comedians called Maddie and Louise, an eighty-two-year-old stand-up called Lynne-Ruth and a handsome Jewish lad named Ben, who was performing a melancholy clowning show. All of us had come from north-west London, yet met in Edinburgh – which is the perfect analogy for how unbearable the Edinburgh festival can be!

But I loved it. I felt like I had come into my own. I slept on strangers' sofas, kitchen floors or, rather intimately, spooned with Louise, because, for the first time in my life, with a new-found confidence, I had introduced myself to a bunch of new people as a gay man.

It turned out that the bar directly next to the pub we'd been performing in happened to be the second biggest gay club in Edinburgh (out of three). So, naturally, one night we all got dolled up, I sprayed some CK One down my pants and made bloody sure that nobody had a concealed cake knife in their clutch bag. Off we all went on my very first night out in a Scottish gay discotheque!

The club was called GHQ, which stood for 'gay headquarters', but from the outside it looked and felt more like 'God hates queers... don't walk outside here after 6pm'. But once I entered GHQ, it was a much friendlier vibe.

I wore a white shirt that was far too small, blue jeans that were tight round the arse and a pair of black boots – I was, frankly, one burgundy lanyard away from a job in Pret. We got wristbands on entry and I wandered around the club to get my bearings, very quickly realising that there were some rooms which I daren't go in ... dark rooms. For any heterosexuals reading, dark rooms are cruising rooms in gay clubs where everything is pitch black except for one ominous flickering red light in a corner, which faintly show the outlines of men having a 'right go on each other', so to speak. (I've only ever entered one of these dark rooms once in my life, feeling someone's hand slide along my upper thigh and my reflexes presumed they were trying to squeeze out and steal my cracked iPhone 5c from my pocket. I'm guessing they were probably trying to squeeze something else.)

On the main dance floor of GHQ I was soon approached by a man in a leather harness, who offered me a little something called poppers. I was immediately suspicious of him, as he was wearing Crocs. Crocs in a gay club is a bold statement, usually suggesting you're either single and still live with your mum or you're an outlandish Central St Martins fashion student with a point to prove.

I told harness man, 'Sorry, I don't do drugs!'

He replied in a thick Glaswegian accent, 'Well they're not *drugs* drugs!'

And so he passed me this bottle, saying 'Liquid Gold', which I stared at, contemplating what to do. All of a sudden I thought, 'Fuck it! I'm in Scotland. No one knows me. Try some poppers!'

And so I opened the lid, raised the open bottle up to my face and took one giant ... swig!

I thought you drank poppers!!

Leather harness man thankfully and aggressively whacked the bottle out of my hand as soon as it touched my lips to prevent me swallowing any amyl nitrate. He then continued to check that I was OK whilst also screaming at me with sheer Scottish fury.

'Wot tae fuck are yah dooin, man?! Aye yoor sueycidal, son?'

After the poppers faux pas I headed to the bar to stick purely to the consumption of spiced rum and Diet Pepsi (they didn't have Diet Coke, which is homophobic in of itself). Whilst I was stood at the bar, this very cute hairy Scottish lad came up to me – let's call him Braveheart for brevity. He had a 20 quid note in his hand and fortunately he was not wearing Crocs.

Braveheart leaned over and said to me, 'Hey, my friend over there thinks you're cute, do you wanna come over for a drink?'

He pointed to a table of trendy-looking bear blokes all wearing fleeces, and gorgeous queer women, also all wearing fleeces, and so I thought, 'Fuck it!'

I popped to the toilet, tucked my shirt in, checked my hair and got spritzed with even more CK One by a toilet attendant, who I believe may have been sat reading the Bible. She then patted me on the back, delivered a quote from the New Testament, and sent me on my way, as is the kindness of thy Christian gay-club-working-neighbour! I gave her a £2 coin, headed over to Braveheart's table and then he came up and said to me, 'Oh, my friend … she's now over there, dancing.'

And I looked over, saw this woman in a fleece dancing and I thought, '*She*? Errrm. OK. I *could* kiss a *she*?!'

And then Braveheart grabbed my arm, stared at my newly turned nineteen-year-old face, assessed the contours of my cheekbones, the presence of mild bum fluff facial hair, and then lent in towards me and said in a tone of clarification, 'You are a lesbian, right?!'

My eyes popped out. Braveheart and I just stared at each other and as I shook my head to suggest a 'No, not a woman!' I watched my masculinity dawn on him, all the wrinkles in Braveheart's forehead shrinking into confusion, then realisation and then finally remorse. It was hilarious.

He overly apologised, which made matters worse. I kindly told him that I wasn't upset and I didn't care. Which I didn't. I didn't care that I'd been mistaken for a lesbian. I'd never care if I was mistaken for a female. To be honest, it happened quite a lot during my teenage years. Male waiters or shopkeepers had often called me 'madam', and older Scottish men in cafés that month had addressed me as 'lassie'. I found it funny when they'd respond with shock or silence upon realising I wasn't female. But I'd rarely give it a second thought, because I just didn't give a shit. It's all a load of bollocks anyway. (Not literally.)

However, being mistaken for a lesbian in a gay club, whilst amusing because I was in a space where I was actively trying to attract myself to people of the same sex, did slightly launch a paranoia in me. Not because I was feminine-looking or anything like that, but because, as a gay man, I didn't look like Braveheart. I didn't really look like what everyone told me was an attractive gay man. I'd often hear straight female friends fantasise over certain gay men and how it was 'such a shame he's gay because he's so gorgeous'. I was never really described as 'gorgeous' or 'fabulous', it was always 'funny' and 'charming'.

Still, to this day, I do not look like 99.9 per cent of the gay men pictured in *Attitude* or *Gay Times* magazine. I'm not one of the muscly, white, oiled guys you see dramatically engaged in a forbidden kiss on the poster for a gay film, gay play or pretty much a gay cultural anything. I think every play written about gay men has had the EXACT same poster concept since plays began.

Instead I was, and still am, a chubby and baby-faced gay man, and this definitely has brought up some insecurities in me – ones I've heard many other gay men and queer friends, regardless of their gender, mention that they struggle with too.

However, before I *fully* get the mini-violin out, I feel it is important to say that, like most things that are cultural phenomena, this image is crafted; it's makebelieve, built around something that's deemed as profitable, with mainstream appeal, but isn't necessarily true or indicative of reality. Or what people actually find attractive.

After I left GHQ, Braveheart bought me a battered sausage supper (which in Scotland involves proper thick-cut chip shop chips and not one but TWO sausages, which is why I'd like Scottish citizenship should they ever attain independence). Then I ended up going back to his place.

And, despite what any gay magazines choose to plug as sexy, if you handle a potentially embarrassing situation by making it funny or charming, perhaps also singing to Lady Gaga's 'Edge of Glory' on a dance floor with pitch-perfect precision, then someone will take you back to theirs for some fun. And they'll be VERY LUCKY to do so.

how to survive your first gay club visit*

(*if someone's gay, straight or any bloody persuasion they damn well wanna be.)

Occasionally I will see people on Twitter describing certain gay clubs that I've felt really uncomfortable in as 'safe spaces' and I'm just like, 'Mate, a safe space is a Caffè Nero without a queue!' Now, I obviously don't want to make sweeping generalisations about *all* gay clubs, but some of them, on a first visit, can feel very intimidating. But, over time, they may become less so.

Straight people can just meet in the Shell garage and – bam – they've got twins and a mortgage the year after. I'm not saying that gays can't do this too, but, there are just fewer neutral places for us to meet and feel comfortable or accepted in that are easily accessible environments. (That, and also gays don't drive! Just remember that. No gay person has ever mastered the forward acceleration of a vehicle. Gays are born not to drive but to be driven. Or so I tell my mum and her Toyota.)

I am also conscious that I'm littering this advice section with disclaimers, because I don't want to scare anyone off or heighten anyone's potential anxieties about going to gay clubs – they can be incredibly fun, but I would recommend also researching things like LGBTQ+ community centres, meet-ups, support groups, queer book shops, etc. These can be great if you or someone you feel is struggling with their sexuality wants to meet other LGBTQ+ people on more neutral turf. And, by neutral, I just mean spaces without bars that may feel less driven by the idea of getting pissed or taking the odd drug. Sadly, we don't have many of these neutral queer spaces in Britain, but there are some if you do the research and I very much hope they are on the rise.

In my early twenties, I often went to gay clubs on my own, as I didn't have many gay pals to go with. Some of these clubs could quite easily make me feel lost and lonely and like I didn't fit in. A lot of this was because of my own insecurities and the conditioning I'd had about how to behave in those places. So here are my tips on how to survive and thrive when first entering the gay bar/clubbing scene:

1 Plan ahead.

Gay bars and gay clubs are all completely different, with varied clientele, themes and general vibes. So do some research and read online and think about what sort of club you might want to go to. Would you prefer a queer cabaret-type space with drag acts and performance at the heart of it, or a club to dance and go on the pull? Gays really love to review shit online, so, honestly, if you want to know if a certain gay club, or branch of Pret or energy provider is any good, just google or tweet search it and you're sure to find some opinionated queers that have written up their personal experiences in detail with a rating out of 10.

2 Don't be judgemental.

This is really important, because you may go into a gay club where you see certain stuff for the very first time that might blow your mind or be different to what you're into.

A lot of clubs are welcoming of people with certain kinks, in certain outfits, or with certain expressions of their gender or sexual identity and the coolest thing you can do is be totally cool with it. If you find it a bit weird, just remember that it doesn't harm you. If you find it really, really weird, then remember that one day you may rather like it. I never thought five years ago that I'd be into Charli XCX, and here I am, writing this at the end of 2019, when, according to Spotify, I've streamed her hundreds of times like a clichéd Twitter gay.

In some gay clubs, certainly the mostly male orientated places I've been into, there may be dark rooms and cruising spots. Don't be a dick about these, don't go round with your iPhone torch on, don't go shouting your friend's name, don't scream about how it kind of smells of poo (these are all things me and my friends have done as naïve, annoying gay boys in dark rooms). If you don't like it then don't go in. If you do like it, then have some fun – but this does bring me on to my next point.

3 Practise and understand consent.
This is 100 per cent relevant for straight clubs too: know not to touch what you shouldn't touch if a signal hasn't been given. Also know that, if someone gropes you and you don't want to be groped, then you have every right to tell them to stop it whenever you want. It doesn't matter if someone's pissed or off their face on a drug of any sort, we have to respect each other. I wish I'd been more forthright and signalled to guys who grabbed parts of me that they shouldn't have.

4 Know your worth.
Gay clubs can (emphasis on 'can') feel like such hyper sexualised places where your character and preferences can often be swept aside by someone's sexually driven behaviour. This is not what me or Lizzo wants for you, so please know your worth. Know you aren't just a vagina or a penis or a bumhole, you're a human being with a family, a personality and, most likely, a more fruitful Boots Advantage card than mine.

Also, I would really recommended not comparing yourself to other people in these spaces. By this I mean that, if someone's boasting they have a ten-inch dick, then they're probably lying. If they're not, tell them to call me!

I'm joking! Obviously – just wish them well like you would if they had a two-inch dick. Two or ten, we're all valid in the club, baby!

5 **Try not to be intimidated.**
Now, I've said loads of stuff that could feel anxiety inducing, but gay clubs are supposed to be fun, accepting, tolerant and inclusive places – so just remember that.

So much of our mainstream gay media/culture can feel about celebrating muscly guys with Johnson's baby oil drizzled over them like a shit salad dressing and so, as I said in the previous chapter, it can be so easy if you don't look like that to feel you don't fit in or that you're in the wrong place. I have found that just because someone looks super stacked and muscly, doesn't mean they aren't just as insecure as a chubby gay guy and haven't just filled in their anxieties with an unhealthy gym addiction. Essentially, we all feel inadequate at times and I think gay clubs are much nicer places when people just chat and get to know one another, and find common ground, regardless of if they're giving someone the glad-eye.

6 **Make sure you hit up the smoking area.**
I do not smoke. In the year 2000, aged six, I was part of something called ITV's Year of the Promise, where 25,000 Britons made a pledge to promise they'd do something for the next millennium. I was one of the youngest to be selected and I have my pledge immortalised on a plaque outside the Greenwich Mean Time museum. This plaque says:

Jack Rooke aged six – 'I promise my dad that I will never ever smoke a cigarette.'

I am very proud to say that twenty years on, I have kept that promise.[1]

However, I do love spending some time in the smoking area. This is usually because, in some clubs, it's the quietest place to chat to someone and it's also where all the best characters are. I guarantee you will hear some top quality anecdotes in the smoking area of any decent gay club. The smoking area is a stage and its performers are nicotine addicts. If you don't smoke, like me, you could fake a vape or stick a Tipp-Ex pen between your fingers, or just proudly say you wanted some air. But do give it a visit!

7 Make friends with the toilet attendant.

This isn't a crucial survival tip; just, in my experience, they tend to be great fun allies in a gay club, like trained psychotherapists lingering round the shitters. They will tell you who is a horrible sleazy regular you should avoid copping off with, as well as tell you if you've got sick/fluff/cum/a phone number written on a receipt stuck in your hair, so do check in on the attendant and they'll do you good, I promise.

8 Feel free to use a dating/hook-up app in the club.

I really believe that, if you're there on your own, it's important to know that other people may be there on

---

[1]   Roll-ups and joints do not count as cigarettes, so, technically, I've kept my pledge.

their own too, and starting a conversation via an app that tells you someone is 83 metres away can sometimes feel much easier and less scary than walking up to someone and saying they look fit/fun/interesting. So I always advise dropping someone a message and arranging to maybe meet up in the club, to take that initial anxiety away.

9 Always thank the bouncer when you're leaving.
This is a suggestion added by my friend Mike, which he swears by. Making pals with the bouncer will stand you in good stead for when you turn up to the club next time and you're completely shit-faced but it is the last place open. Flatter your allies and they'll let you in.

These are tips for you or for you to impart to any nervous gay or questioning pals. I should say that, as I'm writing this book at the ripe old age of twenty-five, which in gay years can feel like seventy-two, I do feel much less intimidated going into most of these places out. I see a lot more new gay adults, six or seven years younger than me, who, on the whole, are living the most accepted queer lifestyles we've ever had in this country. A lot of gay clubs now are places that I hope won't have to always be fuelled by debauched behaviour, but can become a place where queer people can just meet, share stories and be friends, whether you're out on the pull or not.

P.S. If you're in my hometown of London on a night out, the Royal Vauxhall Tavern or The Glory are my personal favourite haunts.

the Olympically gay summer of 2012 – part two

September 2012

A couple days after the Braveheart night at GHQ, I finally had to leave Edinburgh to go back home to London. As I got on the train, I looked on Facebook and saw the news. Jack Groves had taken his own life.

Jack was the guy I'd played 'Never Have I Ever' with eleven months previously during freshers' week and, ironically, we had initially bonded over being the only two men who were 'straight' and hadn't kissed someone of the same sex.

I was so shocked and saddened to hear he'd passed away. That whole summer had been bookended by two young male suicides; two nineteen-year-old boys had taken their own lives in the summer I had also turned nineteen. It made the idea of doing more work and volunteering with CALM feel even more important.

A few weeks later I was at Bestival – this time I got a job hosting the arts stage for the weekend. My best friend Lewis came along too, mainly because Stevie Wonder was headlining and we are OBSESSED! On the Saturday, I snuck off for an hour from my hosting duties to see if I could discover Mr Wonder's dressing room, when all of a sudden I bumped into Brendan – Jack Groves' friend from college, who was on my journalism course. I'd never really changed my preconceived ideas of him as a sort of pretentious, dicky indie boy during that first year at university. But we started chatting and, when it was just me and him in a field full of strangers, we got on quite well. He meandered around some food stalls with me until I just suddenly spurted out, 'I'm so, so sorry about Jack Groves. I know you were friends.'

He told me it had been quite a shock and it was clear he was devastated about it.

We spent my whole afternoon off chatting and seeing some bands together. A character comedy act called Guilt N Shame were performing on the arts stage at 5pm and I was supposed to be back in time to introduce them to the crowd, but me and Brendan were having such a good chat that I just completely forgot. We swapped numbers, agreed to have a drink when we started second year. I felt so awful

I had concocted such a terrible impression of Brendan. He actually wasn't the prick, I was!

I went back to my stage at 5.45pm and gave a grovelling apology to the two guys who performed in Guilt N Shame, Gabe and Rob. It turned out they didn't give a shit. To make up for it, the following day they did their show again and I introduced them to a packed-out, overly excited amphitheatre of festival revellers desperate for some comedy ahead of Stevie's headline set. The Guilt N Shame show was all about a gay guy and a straight guy who were best mates, getting up to all sorts of trouble and ribbing each other for their shortcomings.

And whether or not I was inspired by these silly characters, or just the whole summer I'd had, that night, after we'd watched HRH Stevie Wonder on the main stage, I took Lewis to sit on the top of a hill to watch the fireworks of Bestival 2012. It was here that I told him I was gay. I explained how I'd fallen for Nick Mathieson earlier in the year, had my heart broken and was finally, for the first time since Dad died, starting to feel like myself. I had started to like who I was becoming after trying to conceal so much of myself for so long.

Lewis smiled, said he didn't care, and instead of taking half a tab of acid and subsequently shitting ourselves, we went and got a cup of tea at the Women's Institute tent.

That was the end of my first gay summer. It had involved kissing a boy by a tree who left me to kiss another boy by a tree, ripping out someone's septum piercing whilst trying to fellate them, nearly drinking from a bottle of poppers and then being mistaken for a lesbian whilst on the pull in a gay club. I wish these stories were hyperbolic for dramatic effect, but they are all, very sadly, painfully true. And, after spending all summer relishing the anonymity that being in new places had given me, it ended with me, sat telling someone who I'd known my whole life about who I really was.

how to tell a friend about your sexuality

I know I did an advice bit on how to support someone who's in the process of accepting their sexuality and how to really listen to that person properly. However, I also think it's just as important to come out to people properly too. By 'properly', I don't mean you have to give them a set-in-concrete definition of your sexuality, quite the opposite really. Though I do think it's important to be transparent with someone you love who you want to know the truth about you.

1 It might be a good idea to start by explaining why you haven't discussed or told them about your sexuality before. There are so many complex reasons for this and whatever yours is, it is completely valid. Everything with regards to talking about one's sexuality needs to be on the watch of the person trying to figure theirs out.

2 I think it's good to lay out what you might want someone to do to help you, whether that be big, small or nothing at all, and for everything to remain as normal.

Cecilia was one of the first people I told I was gay, mainly because I just wanted to come out to someone who I knew had already loved and accepted someone who was gay. Despite how utterly tragic it is that her brother Leo is no longer here, I felt so inspired by how Cecilia dealt with it. How she wanted to talk about him always, how she was protective of him and wanted to for ever remember his little camp, flamboyant idiosyncrasies, whilst also understanding the internally homophobic tendencies he had, some of which I could really understand and empathise with.

I think, for me, whilst I hate the term 'coming out', and disagree with the idea that anyone should have to, for me the one important thing about coming out to someone is them essentially saying: I want you to protect me. I want you to understand me and accept me no matter what.

If, for whatever reason, someone doesn't accept someone else's confidence in their sexuality as a good or positive thing, then they at least need to accept that someone has the right to be anyone they want.

3 Finally, just be honest. Be protective of yourself and what exactly you want to divulge and try to be kind in response to any silly or confused questions. We are all learning and we all need to be educated about the spectrum of how people live and identify, because, ultimately, that is the truth to being a happy person.

Bakerloo blues

September 2012–March 2013

That autumn I returned to university and moved into my second-year flat, an absolute dive of a four-bed maisonette above a rather beige branch of Santander bank. We affectionately named it 'Santander Palace' – despite finding six dead rats behind the oven on the day we moved in.

The flat was in a relatively small neighbourhood in the outer north-west London suburbs called Kenton, which, I'm afraid, was a total shit-hole. And not a loved one. Upon moving there, my Aunty Jenny described Kenton as 'A great place if you're looking for cheap dentistry', which I think paints quite an accurate picture of what a beige town it was. To make matters worse, Kenton was only served by Bakerloo Line trains and, as anyone who has lived in or visited London will probably be able to tell you, the Bakerloo Line is the worst line if you ever want to get somewhere, which is predominantly what I was trying to use it for.

As I started my second year, Olly was entering his third, and he had very sweetly chosen me to take over his role as head of news at the student radio station. Because of this, we had to do a series of handover sessions, during which it became clear that we'd now gone from 'third year mentoring second year' to becoming actual friends.

He asked me about the poetry gigs I'd done over the summer and we agreed that we'd go to some nights together. Soon enough, Olly came with me when I performed at Bang Said the Gun, the stand-up poetry gig I'd been invited to perform at after the Brighton festival slam. This night took place above a pub in London Bridge and, after doing a couple fun, well-received gigs there, the guys who ran the night asked if I would like to start hosting it as a resident compere, which I excitedly agreed to. Unlike most poetry nights, Bang Said the Gun was fun because it played host to a mix of poets, comedians and storytellers. I'd be introducing headline acts from Scroobius Pip and Kate Tempest to Josie Long and Howard Marks. It was a dream gig!

Once I'd started hosting, Olly came even more regularly to the gigs with me, bringing his flatmate, Claire, who was also studying at our uni in his year. Claire became a good pal of mine – an honest, frank, funny, stunning and very sweet Northerner who would put you in your place with one glance if you were being a dickhead. Which is, quite frankly, an essential characteristic in any friendship group.

The two of them would sit in the front row of the audience on a finger-hole-picked red leather Chesterfield and be my audience hype girls for the night. I'd often catch Olly's eye as he absorbed the atmosphere – grinning at people's silly poems with a can of Red Stripe in hand. Sometimes I'd feel bittersweet pangs of grief that my dad would never be in the audience. He would have loved these nights of bizarre absurdist humour. But the whole experience of hosting it every week gave me back so much of the confidence that I'd lost as a teenager.

After the headline acts, we'd have an open mic section, and each week Olly would threaten to sign up for a slot to read some of his own poems. Then he would chicken out or be a no-show and not tell anyone why. I started noticing this behaviour quite early on in our friendship – a sort of panic that would set into him. It was an insecurity of sorts, which felt in conflict with how charming and bold he could be.

Meanwhile, at university in the first semester of my second year, my course project was to start a new magazine, creating, producing, writing and designing it with a group of other students. My friend Tom was the editor; he picked me and Brendan to be culture writers and a girl called Lily to be the designer. Lily had deferred a year and had just come back to her studies, so she had been in the year above and knew Olly very well. And this project was an absolute blast. After our time at Bestival, Brendan and I had massively warmed to each other and now we really hit it off.

Looking back, it's quite strange that after such a gay-orientated summer, I came back for second year and became best mates with two straight lads, but both Olly and Brendan were just so fun. They had infectious energies to be around, like when you meet someone and find yourself fizzing around them, giddy with immaturity and naivety, like kids in a seaside sweet shop. However, both Olly and Brendan also had their own struggles, just like I did, and whilst you couldn't see them on the surface of our behaviour, all three of us were trying to overcome them.

Brendan lived with his brother here in a small flat above a pub. Most people I knew at our university lived with friends above a pub in north London, but Brendan was a 47-minute tube ride away. When I first went round his with some mates he spewed out a number of disclaimers about it, which is usually a sign that someone's in an odd living situation.

'So there's only one bedroom and it's not mine and it's quite dirty right now, but we can all just chill in the living room.'

The flat was fine but quite cramped. Jordan's brother had the one bedroom whilst Brendan slept in the living room on a tiny single bed in the corner. I remember seeing that Brendan kept Jack's funeral pamphlet Blu-Tacked right next to his bed. I can remember doing this with my dad's.

I visited Jordan's flat a couple times over the next few months whilst we were working on our magazine project together. Over pints, Brendan told me about his upbringing and some of the difficulties, of which it's not my right to divulge in a book, but what I *can* say is that neither of us had had the easiest of teenage years. We'd both had absent people in our lives for different reasons.

It was clear that Brendan wasn't happy in this flat. One morning after a big night out when I slept on his floor, I remember asking him some questions about Jack Groves and he burst into tears. I didn't know whether or not to hug him. I wanted to, and to tell him everything was all right, but I wasn't sure if that's what Brendan wanted or needed. He asked me if it was weird that he still sometimes spoke to Jack, chatted to him in his head when he was on his own. I told Brendan how I used to actually ring my dad's phone number for maybe twelve weeks after he died, leaving him voicemails, sometimes crying and asking for him to come home. (Eventually my mum decided we could put the money we were spending on a dead man's phone contract towards getting Sky Plus, which was a plan I was very much down for.) But when my dad's number was cut, when it became a three-beep 'this number is not in use', my heart really broke. I had called him every day as a kid, I knew his phone number like my birthday, and I always wanted so desperately to just call him one more time. I understood how, for Brendan also, it is so hard to detach yourself from having conversations with someone you've lost so suddenly.

Soon I came to realise that where Brendan was living wasn't somewhere you could properly grieve. It wasn't somewhere he could have his own space and privacy. I thought about how, in my first year of grief, my mum had kept our house as loving and warm as it was before and that was such safety to me. I knew that was what Brendan needed. He needed somewhere that was his.

So, with Brendan unhappy in his living situation, me detesting living in Kenton and my pal Lewis being sick of living with his parents in suburbia, we all decided, after a few pub nights out, that we'd find somewhere to move into together. Within minutes of dreaming up this plan, I was assigned Zoopla, Brendan was assigned RightMove.com and Lewis was assigned to ask his rich dad if he could be all of our guarantors.

We decided to focus our search around north-west London's Kilburn and West Hampstead, because this area was near to where Olly and Claire lived and, essentially, because we loved the pubs around there. At nineteen years old, that was a good enough reason around which to base our *Location Location Location* property search.

Soon enough we found a flat, signed the contracts and had a moving-in date. This was it!

how to know if a friend is the right person to move in with

It's really hard to strike the right balance of characters when moving in with friends and, as I said, if you're going through a hard time, then it's so important to have a living space that keeps you sane. Somewhere that feels safe and homely, and also somewhere that helps quell any anxieties rather than exacerbate them. And living with others means you need to understand and get on board with people's anxieties, tendencies, behaviours, shopping habits, weird quirks and alarm songs. This was something I soon realised.

My alarm song was a rather abrasive M.I.A. album track called 'Meds and Feds'. If you want to, YouTube search this song and listen to the first 45 seconds and imagine what it was like to hear someone in the bedroom next door waking up to that song every day. I have driven numerous friends of mine mad over the years through having to hear it but, for about two years, those opening guitar riffs used to really kick me into gear each morning.

Now, this advice section doesn't fully relate to mental health or wellbeing tips as such. I just always think who you're living with and where are good things to properly think about, because it will have an impact on your state of mind. You want to live with friends who you can laugh, cry with and talk to about a shit date you'd just had at 3am whilst holding cups of decaff tea. It's got to be someone whose hair you don't mind fishing out the plughole on occasion. Or someone you can spontaneously have a takeaway with and trust they will actually pay you back, or will take it in turns.

I guess the answer to this question is that you never really know if someone's right to live with until you do, but I really believe that people should think long and hard over it and what impact a new living situation will have on them.

Despite having this weird irrational dislike of Brendan in first year, by my second year I was suddenly moving in with him and it was one of the best things I ever did for my wellbeing, because he was exactly that person I could have a laugh with but also chat to whenever each other felt down.

the pubs of
Kilburn –
part one

March–April 2013

We got the keys for our new flat on Olly's twenty-sixth
birthday, with just enough time to get all our stuff moved in
and then get ourselves out of the flat and on the piss. It was
a level of foolproof recklessness that I would never possess
the stamina to partake in nowadays.

Our flat was a fairly basic but a nice enough two-bed,
part of an old Victorian house in West Hampstead with high
ceilings and two toilets – the dream property for nineteen-
year-old me and my occasional dalliances (flare-ups) with
IBS. The only downside was – there were three of us. But
getting a two-bed flat was the only way we could afford to
live somewhere fancy enough to feel a million miles away

from the depressive landscape of Kenton and be as close as we could be to central London.

I lived in a back room, right down the end of a long winding corridor and down some steps. It transpired it was an extension on to the house, which we realised when a giant crack formed next to my bedroom door and a surveyor said – in technical terms I can't remember – that my room was falling off the house. This was the price we paid for Zone Two life – the potential for my living quarters to cave and collapse inwards.

Brendan took the middle bedroom in between me and Lewis. I initially suggested this because it felt weirdly important that, as me and Lewis had been best friends for the best part of twenty years, Brendan was physically in the middle of us and knew we were both there for him. Ultimately, though, Brendan didn't give a single shit.

And, finally, poor Lewis lived in a door-less but massive living room, on a sofa-bed which he threw a king-size matt-ress on top of. We fixed a huge red velvet curtain to a pole that he could pull over the hallway to have some semblance of privacy, though he occasionally had to deal with a drunk me wandering into his room at 3am and getting into bed with him, demanding we watch an episode of *Summer Heights High*. Weirdly, Lewis never really complained about this, which is ironic, because, had I been him, I would've turned into a Medusa-like creature spitting fury on anyone who passed that iron curtain.

And so, once we were all settled in, we went off for drinks at the North London Tavern in Kilburn, where our friend Tom from our magazine project worked behind the bar. We met up with Olly and Claire, who were just up the hill in Cricklewood, and got a house-warming round in.

Five drinks in, me and Olly stood, tipsy, at the bar, ordering another pint of Red Stripe for him and a diabetically sweet strawberry-and-lime cider for me. He rolled his eyes at my drinks choices and then asked me if I thought the barmaid was fit.

I replied, 'Oh … yeah! Hell YEAH she is!!'

Olly still didn't know I liked boys. The fruity cider hadn't been enough of a clue. It wasn't something we had ever spoken about and so I'd just left it. And then, after we were served our drinks, he dragged me off into the disabled loo for a chat, locked the door and sat me on the toilet. He lifted down the baby changing unit, wiping it with some wet tissues, drying it with some dry tissues and then he started racking up, all these lines of, let's say 'white powdered poetry'.

Soon enough, there were five lines of 'white poetry' on a changing unit, which I pointed out to Olly would typically be covered in baby shit, but he proclaimed that he'd cleaned it sufficiently enough. And then, one by one, random people from the bar who knew Olly just walked in, 'did some lines of poetry' and left. It was like a conveyor belt of 'poetry' and I just sat there, watching it all unfold with my pint of fruity cider until there was only one line of prose left.

Olly said, 'For you?'

I replied, 'Nah, I don't really do that sort of poetry.'

And then he said, without forcing me or peer pressuring me, 'But have you ever even done *this* sort of poetry?'

And I said, 'No, I've never done coke!'

He laughed, licked his finger, swiped up the line and said he could just rub a tiny bit of poetry all over my gums and it would just give me a little pick-up for a couple of hours. And for some reason, in the excitement of the moment, and having just moved to a brand new place in a brand new town starting a brand new chapter of my life, I nodded.

'When you first dragged me in the bogs with you I didn't think this is what you wanted to put in my mouth!'

Olly chuckled, 'Naughty Jacky!', and then told me to shut up as he grabbed my jaw and started rubbing some poetry all around the inner cavity of my gob.

'Olly, it tastes fucking disgusting!'

'So does strawberry-and-lime cider, mate.'

We left the loo and all of a sudden I just reeeaaaalllly wanted to chat. Like reeeeaaaaaalllllllllyyyyyyyy wanted a good old natter about life.

Imagine that, some 'poetry' making two gobshite uni students want to have a DMC (deep meaningful conversation). It's almost too clichéd to publish in a book.

In this DMC, I vaguely remember telling Olly that, for a few years after Dad died, I avoided going into pubs because, after spending time in them with him as a kid, sometimes pubs would remind me how much I missed him, how much I longed to see him sat on a bar stool with a pint of Kronenbourg, getting his false teeth plate out to show the bar staff.

Olly told me about his dad, explaining that he left the UK, moved to Japan and has got a new family out there. He told me how he loves to visit them, showing me photos of his siblings.

And then Olly said, quite casually in this chat, that he was on medication for 'up there', tapping his head like that infamous gif meme of Roll Safe in *Hood Documentary*, as if he'd come up with an idea. He told me that sometimes he gets really depressed, but right now he was pretty happy.

To lighten the mood, we spoke about happiness. I tried to explain that, for me, happiness is when you walk into an Asda you've never been to before and you see it's got two floors. (This is a particularly niche thing I enjoy, which I weirdly found myself quite passionate about whilst on 'lines of poetry'.)

We laughed, and Olly said that ultimate happiness for him was a Newcastle United win and a good old dance.

'Dancing?' I said.

He smiled. 'Dancing!'

So Olly and I snuck off without saying goodbye to anyone, across the road to Powers bar – a sort of gentrified artsy haunt with dangly lightbulbs you could get a brain injury from, where the barmaids all looked like Laura Marling and a relatively crap DJ stood in the corner playing off-kilter swing/indie music.

All of a sudden in this bar I was just buzzing, improvising dance moves on the spot, because that's what 'poetry' does to me. Olly got us in two piña coladas and said, 'Jack, you are a fabulous dancer!'

From this night onwards the little group from our move-in night out started meeting up twice weekly at different happy hours along or around Kilburn High Road. We often finished our Friday nights at a pub called the Good Ship, for their 'indie-disco' night. One Friday, the whole gang was storming down the high street to join the back of the queue to get in, when me and Olly realised we didn't have cash for entry. Just us two left to go and get cash and it was at the ATM outside Brondesbury train station that I nervously, finally, after months of waiting, told Olly that, 'I fancy men!'

There was a slight drunken pause, as he turned to me nonchalantly and said, 'Jack, you're like my brother, why would I give a fuck you big ol' poof? Get £20 out quickly, or else it's more expensive to get in after midnight!'

I smiled and told him off for using that word. He apologised and said it was only out of love. In the queue Olly then asked if I could tie my hair into a bun, so he could put a 'baggy of poetry' in it and, naturally, I obliged – security guards never check eighteen-stone gay guys' man buns.

We got our hands stamped, found everyone else and danced all night long. When M.I.A.'s 'Paper Planes' came on in the club, Olly lifted me off the ground as everyone crowded round me, singing it in my face like a football chant. These nights out with this group of friends were honestly some of the happiest times of my life. Things were still tough, but I was coping and I felt like I belonged.

At the end of a night out, friends would often come back to our flat and get more pissed, drifting off in dribs and drabs. One night I told Olly he could just stay in my room and he said, 'Yeah, OK then!' before flopping on to my floor.

I said he could just stay in my bed with me, but he said he was happy on the floor with a blanket.

I replied, 'Come off it, I'm not trying to shag you, you might be six years older than me, but you're still too young for me!'

And Olly stubbornly said, 'No, down here is fine.'

And then we fell asleep.

The next morning when I woke up, I realised he'd got into bed with me, top to tail, like teenagers having a school sleepover.

the pubs of Kilburn – part two

One night we were at a pub called The Betsy Smith at the bottom of Kilburn High Road. I'm telling this story because it was when Olly first said that he'd thought in the past about suicide. He'd had those pangs of suicidal ideation which many people with mental health issues can experience at times. Statistics suggest that around one in five of us will have had these thoughts at least once in our lifetimes.

But, back then, in our semi-drunken chat, I quite naively and almost nonchalantly challenged Olly on this: 'Why? Why would you ever do that? You're clever, you're funny, you're fit – like why would you do that? Why would you leave us?'

And Olly leaned in and said with such a bizarre sense of clarity, 'Mate, I wouldn't ever want to leave you, I'd want to leave me.'

I didn't know how to respond, unsure what I could possibly say to something so heartbreaking. I guess that conversation sowed a seed in my mind that, one day, if he really was vulnerable enough, he could do it.

As I said in the introduction to this book, I think we all know someone who we have a similar low-key worry about. Not necessarily that they'd take their own life, but that they have a sadness about them, a vulnerability which could be damaging to themselves. I occasionally worried about Olly and how he could be very sensitive and erratic, but I didn't know what I personally could do. Nowadays I think that all you can do in that situation is just remind someone they are loved and that help is available out there.

It was on this night that I started to tell Olly about my friend Cecilia and her brother Leo. I told him that me and Cecilia had become ambassadors of the charity CALM over the summer and that we were starting to put on fundraising gigs for them. These shows were called 'Save the Male', after a campaign that CALM was running at the time to raise awareness of suicide as the single biggest killer of young men. Cecilia and I wanted to promote creativity as an outlet and as a form of catharsis to help more young men to figure stuff out in their heads, so the night was a mix of comedy, poetry, performance art, rap and just general storytelling – as many different creative disciplines as we could cram into one line-up.

Inspired by this, Olly then put his own fundraiser on – a poetry and music night at a local library arts space. My poetry collective headlined it and I'm very glad to say that, by this point, I had fully given up on the awful Madeleine McCann poem and was writing much funnier material!

Putting on his fundraiser gave Olly the confidence to realise he should finally try out performing, and stop dropping out of the Bang Said the Gun open mic. So one night whilst I was hosting, he nervously plucked up the courage to perform.

Now, the open mic slam at Bang Said the Gun could either be brilliant or terrible. It tended to depend on what sort of people we'd get signing up. It could either be those studying English Lit at Goldsmiths and copying Kate Tempest's accent for two minutes whilst doing a poem about love, or it could be someone in their late seventies doing something completely, authentically brilliant. One week I told Olly, in a tough love tone, that he *HAD* to do it. He agreed.

Watching Olly becoming anxious before this performance was hard, because you could see all his bravado drain away as he became a shell-like nervous shadow of himself, terrified of maybe getting it wrong or feeling humiliated. I recognised those anxious symptoms – I'd experienced them, too, but somehow performing had actually helped me. I told him to just take deep breaths and remember it's only two minutes of speaking in front of a very friendly audience.

I introduced Olly to the stage and he took the mic and started reading a poem off his iPhone notes about a girl who stole his chips on a night out. I could see his legs shaking whilst he read and he spoke at almost double speed, nervously spewing out words to get it over with. But as he finished, the audience erupted into applause. He was brilliant, despite the nerves, and I was so proud that he'd finally done it.

He came off stage and said, 'Ooh, I rather enjoyed that!'

And BAM! Our boy was a poet!

As the months went on, he continued to sign up to the odd open mic, his performance style landing somewhere in between Mike Skinner and Danny Dyer. He would HATE me for saying that. I'd love to say in a nostalgic tone that I remember all Olly's poems, but I don't, mainly because some of them were too sophisticated for me and because I was always a bit pissed. But Olly's writing showed how he could really digest the abstract, the pain in lyrics, metaphors that would spin him out into a daze of thoughts. Whereas I just liked dick jokes that rhymed.

Olly wasn't as confident as me, but I remember so vividly, one night after he performed, Olly said to me that I gave him confidence, which, from a straight attractive lad to a fat gay like me, felt like quite the compliment. To give a mate confidence, to help them feel more like themselves is, to my mind, one of the most honoured parts of a true friendship.

One night I was asked by the organisers not to host but to perform my own stuff. I decided I wanted to try some comedy material for the very first time – no grief poems, just funny stuff. Olly came and sat at the front and I started my set with a funny poem called 'Not the One', about realising that I didn't love someone when it transpired they'd never had a chicken katsu curry from Wagamama. And, to finish, I performed a piece about bisexuality, a Katie Melua cover song called '9 Billion Bisexuals in Beijing'. I had ripped an instrumental of the song off YouTube and sang along with my own lyrics:

There are Nine Billion Bisexuals in Beijing
That's a fact!
No one can ever say it's not true –
Lady Gaga, Jessie J, Duncan from Blue

I finished this performance to my first ever standing ovation and, as I came off the stage, Olly ran up to me and gave me the biggest hug. And I will always remember him saying: 'That was you, Jack! That was you on stage. This is what you should do – it was career-defining, you should be so proud. I'm so proud of you.'

I'm welling up as I write this, because these words have never left me. Quite honestly, it was the first time I'd heard the words 'I'm proud of you' said by another man since my dad. Olly was six years older than me and, within eighteen months of becoming friends, I knew I could just speak to him about anything. He looked out for me, and he could dish out the tough love too, in particular calling me out if he thought I was being lazy with work or being consumed by insecurities about my size or appearance. But he would positively reinforce so much about me.

Whilst I knew my mum was proud of me, there was a part of me which honestly just wanted a male figure to say it, to properly look out for me. And I think of the times he told me that I made him feel confident and I wish with all my heart that I had said it back. Because, in many ways, that is exactly what he did for me too.

first gay Pride

July 2013

When you're the only gay in the gang, going to Pride can feel a little lonely. Back in July 2013, I still didn't have many good queer pals I could tag along with, so instead I plucked up the courage to ask some straights. And by 'ask some straights', I mean 'dupe Lewis and Olly into going for a drink in Soho on the day of Pride and then act shocked upon the discovery there were literally thousands of gays there'.

We all walked around, watching big hairy blokes strutting about in PVC straps, with thighs bare but bulges covered in leather. Olly soaked up the spectacle, walking the line of surprised straight man face and laughing along with the flamboyance of it all.

I caught him chatting to an older gay couple outside Caffè Nero on Old Compton Street, and – whether true or not – I felt like he wanted to speak to them to maybe know more about me, and – whether true or not – I felt that they wanted to speak to him to see if he'd sell them any meow meow and have a threesome with them after.

I soon whisked him away to the nearest bar.

We all stood, drunk and dancing to queer pop hits, when, all of a sudden, Lady Gaga's 'Edge of Glory' came on. This was my song. It still is MY song. This is because, from three minutes to four minutes in, there's a saxophone solo from Clarence Clemons, who used to be in Bruce Springsteen's band, and the week the song came out, he passed away and, every time I hear that saxophone solo, it gives me many feels.

As the song came on, Olly also lost his shit and started to tell me how the song is musically and rhythmically one of the best pop songs of our generation, pouring his heart out like an overly keen intern at *NME* magazine. And so we shouted it to each other – that feeling when you sing a song to someone else, when it's just you and them and no one else matters.

Afterwards, I clocked this guy in a T-shirt that said 'Britney Survived 2007 You Can Handle Today'. I quite fancied him. He had the gruff, hairy, bear-like qualities of Eric Cantona crossed with a young, fresh-faced Keir Starmer. Go now and google 'Young Keir Starmer'. Very handsome.

He started moving near us and Olly said to me, 'GET IN THERE, MATE', and so I did. I started dancing with young Keir Starmer.*

---

* Young Keir Starmer definitely seemed far less of a wet wipe than present day Keir Starmer.

I turned back around and realised Olly had gone. Only about 15 minutes had passed and I hadn't seen him leave. It was a behaviour I started to notice more and more, and it wasn't always in a funny Irish-goodbye-at-a-friend's-shithouse-party kind of way, but just a complete disappearing act. No 'I'm off', no text afterwards explaining, nothing. When I asked Olly the next day what happened, he'd just say that he needed to go home and get to bed. It was just one of many little signs that he wasn't always OK. That sometimes his mental health issues affected him in moments where I'd have thought he was happy as Larry.

After trying to find Olly for ten minutes, I then lost Britney T-shirt guy, so me and Lewis just stayed on the dance floor amongst dribs and drabs of half-friends, new acquaintances and the total strangers that you end up rollicking with in a club at Pride.

But it was perhaps the first time I quite seriously realised that I was worried about Olly.

how to spot some early signs of mental health issues in loved ones (and help them to open up and get help)

It can often be those closest to someone who first spot the signs that their behaviour has changed. It's important to understand how not every person who's depressed is moody and not everyone who's anxious looks nervous. The other day, my mum said to me in a panic, 'Oh no, why do you look so sad?' and the only thing wrong was that I really, really needed a poo.

Some of the symptoms of people experiencing a bad period of mental wellbeing may be very well hidden indeed. There are also symptoms that can obviously just be temporary, like feeling stressed or angry about an incident at work or sad because Derek has ghosted you on Tinder. Many of these feelings will hopefully soon pass. However, if they start to seem recurrent, it could be a sign someone is struggling and not finding proper solutions for it.

It's become more and more widely known within the mainstream mental health conversation that one in four people will have some form of mental health problem in their lifetime. However, for as many as 1 in 50, this problem will be serious enough to affect their ability to work or to form stable personal relationships, and this is where we need to feel more able to spot those signs early and offer a helping hand.

Generally, some of the signs I've spotted in some of my friends that I try to speak about are:

- Someone excessively worrying, or always seeming fearful or paranoid about stuff.
- Someone feeling frequently sad or low.
- Someone who you can see is having problems with concentrating or focusing in conversations.
- Someone who isn't really sleeping or feeling like they're functioning properly.
- Someone who is experiencing severe mood changes, including super 'highs'/feelings of euphoria and then absolute 'lows' of sadness or strong feelings of irritability or anger.
- Someone who is actively avoiding their friends and social activities in favour of being more isolated – like Olly leaving nights out early without saying goodbye.

These can all be tough things to watch someone go through, and it can also be easy to mis-read some of these behaviours and feel like maybe you have done something wrong. Generally, though, I'd say it's important if you are worried to flag them. It doesn't mean you are starting some huge intervention or that you need to admit you've been monitoring someone's behaviour, it just means you care and you want to tell someone that you understand they're going through a hard time. Here are some tips on how to do that:

1 Maybe take them for a good walk or somewhere calm and peaceful to chat. Going for a coffee or even suggesting lunch in the park can be a less pressured way to approach speaking to someone about their emotional state. I would recommend avoiding the pub, because alcohol is a depressant, but only you can judge where your friend is most likely to feel safe and ready to open up.

2 I know I've said it millions of times, but make sure you properly listen to what someone tells you when they do open up about their state of mind. Keep back any of your personal judgements and try to be as diplomatic as possible. Look for clues not just in what they are saying, but in what they are *not* saying too, and make sure you stay calm in response to everything they may offload. Remember you are there to be a support and they are going to need you for more than just a one-day walkabout.

The Samaritans publish a method of tips for active listening called SHUSH. These stand for:

S – Show you care. Focus on the other person, make eye contact, put away your phone. To really listen you need to give them your full attention and try not to talk about yourself at all, unless coming up with valid examples of stuff you can empathise with them on.

H – Have Patience. It may take time and several attempts before a person is ready to open up. The person sharing shouldn't feel rushed, or they won't trust or feel that it's a safe environment in which to open up. If they paused in their response, just wait, as they may not have finished speaking. It might take them some time to formulate what they are saying, or they may find it difficult to articulate what they're feeling. You don't need to fill any awkward silences.

U – Use open questions that need more than a yes/no answer, and follow up with questions like 'Could you tell me more?' This also means not jumping in with your own ideas about how the other person may be feeling. Open-ended questions tend not to impose a viewpoint and require a person to pause, think and reflect, and then hopefully expand on how they're feeling.

S – Say it back. I have often found at times, when my anxieties have been incredibly bad, that telling someone and hearing them quite rationally and calmly repeat it back to me can feel really reassuring. It's also a really good way to reassure them that they have your undivided attention.

H – Have courage. Don't be put off by an initial negative response that you might get. Sometimes it can feel intrusive and counter-intuitive to ask someone how they feel, but you'll soon be able to tell if someone is uncomfortable and doesn't want to engage with you at that level.

Source: samaritans.org.

3 If they say that they feel depressed or need help, you could help them make that doctor's appointment phone call. It's estimated that one in three GP appointments fall under the umbrella of mental health care, despite the fact most GPs are trained more in physical illnesses. It's also totally fine for someone to ask for a friend or relative to come into a GP appointment if they are anxious that they won't be able to articulate how they've been feeling or talk about it without bursting into tears.

What will likely happen during this appointment is that the GP will figure out the right course of treatment for someone in need. This might be medication, of which there are different types, such as anti-depressants, mood stabilisers, anti-psychotics and much more, all aiming to help support the brain's functioning to help someone's mental state.

The GP may also opt for a referral for some talking therapy, such as CBT (cognitive behavioural therapy), which can help you manage your problems by changing the way you think and behave. Or there are more relationship-focused therapies, some more suitable for people displaying symptoms of PTSD and so on.

There are so many types of treatment and so much of it is all about trial and error, figuring out the right method and right treatment to best help someone. It is so important as the loved one of someone in this early process that you're there to support them in these times. There may be side effects that don't work for some people, and medications or treatments may change. This is all a normal part of the process.

You may also want to sit and help someone as they fill in the various questionnaires and paperwork that come with accessing treatment, which can feel really stressful at times. I once had to fill in a 'strengths and difficulties' questionnaire to get some free therapy off the NHS and the questionnaire asked me to assign numerical ratings to my feelings and the likelihood that I may take my own life, and I found it really tough. It can be a daunting experience trying to get help, but there is help out there and that's the important thing to remind someone.

I would also say that even if someone says they want to pay for a private therapist for CBT and talking therapies, it's still always good to see a GP first and foremost to flag to them that someone's been struggling for a while.

4 They can also speak to helplines, like the Samaritans 24-hour helpline, or CALM's helpline, which is open most evenings. A text-line mental health service was launched last year, which I found out more about by writing an essay for Scarlett Curtis's brilliant book *It's Not OK To Feel Blue (& Other Lies)*, which was released in conjunction with the charity SHOUT. They run a free anonymous text line for anyone to send messages to trained advisors in times of a struggle.

I'll list lots of these numbers and support lines at the back of the book (see p. 395).

Finally, there may be more severe symptoms you might notice in a loved one, such as self-harm, an over-reliance on alcohol or drugs, or perhaps some worrying comments or behaviour on social media. In these cases I would really recommend reaching out and encouraging your friend to get urgent medical help, depending on the severity of the behaviour. Mental health charities like Samaritans, CALM or MIND can be good to contact as a first port of call and you can also check out a website called 'Befrienders Worldwide', which I discovered through Samaritans, which is a huge directory of helplines for certain mental health issues all across the world.

GPs may be able to contact local early intervention services for mostly under thirty-five-year-old patients, if you believe your friend is showing signs of psychosis, which is when someone's mental state is incredibly vulnerable. A psychotic episode would involve their symptoms starting to include hearing voices or having unusual paranoias or beliefs that may bring harm to themselves, and so it's crucial to get help as soon as possible.

Whether it's something more severe or a period of sustained low mood, it's very important to just encourage someone to seek help and know that there's nothing they can lose by trying to gain more support. We all go through shit times and we all have the ability to get through it with the right care and treatment.

I often think about that T-shirt at Gay Pride which said 'Britney Survived 2007. You Can Handle Today' and, yes, whilst it might be a camp, snappy sentiment for a fashion slogan tee, I do try to remind myself or my loved ones in times of struggle that other people have been in the same place and they have successfully sought help. (Fair enough, Britney's a multi-millionaire, but you know what I mean: there is always more help out there than you think!)

CALM volunteering

Summer 2013

The day Olly got his university results we sat on the green beside the Royal Festival Hall, staring at the London Eye with gins in tins to celebrate. He was one mark off a first and, in typical Olly fashion, he was not having any of it. He appealed to get some modules re-marked and, thankfully, this bumped him up a few marks.

He told me that day to start thinking, before I entered my third year, about my thesis topic and listing potential subject ideas. Journalism BA dissertations are, as you can imagine, all about researching, studying and investigating an area of the media. And, as quite a lot of things in journalism are quite fucked up and problematic, it wasn't too difficult to come up with something.

Around this time, Claire and Olly had left their flat in Cricklewood. Olly was living with some friends and Claire had moved into a property guardianship – which became incredibly popular around this time, as it was one of few ways that skint people could actually live in London's Zones One to Five for an affordable amount. This was almost through legalised squatting in unused, empty buildings. Essentially taking on the role of lodger meets security guard. These buildings could be offices, pubs, schools ... I even have some friends who live in an actual morgue. A MORGUE!

That summer I had to do work experience as part of my degree and I did this at CALM, working with their media department. By media department, I mean the one and only media officer, who was called Rachel. She was an absolute diamond to intern for.

That year, the Samaritans had published a hugely important and influential report acknowledging that a key factor influencing male suicide was the cultural stereotypes that we expect blokes to live up to. CALM was originally set-up and spearheaded by a woman called Jane Powell, an incredible activist, feminist and campaigner, who replied to this report, saying: 'If the fault lies in the culture – not the men – then it is our expectations, stereotypes, and the messages embedded within our daily lives and our media that need to be tackled if we are to have any long-term impact upon male suicide. CALM aims to change this culture, not simply just provide support.'

Jane was incredible, as was Rachel, and what they wanted to achieve was so ambitious that I expected to be doing my work experience in some huge team of charity sector workers, encompassing data analysts, fundraisers, advisors, etc. Instead I rocked up to CALM's office that summer to find just five women in one room that stank of sweaty feet, tucked behind Borough Market, just south of the River Thames. I was astonished that such a growing charity, with a campaign gaining more and more momentum every month, was actually being held together by a small bunch of get-shit-done gals! But of course it was.

I wrote a piece in 2018 for *GQ* about how, actually, lads, we have a lot to thank these women for in terms of increasing awareness of male suicide and that a huge section of that fourth wave of feminism was, in fact, trying to raise awareness of the elements of masculinity that were keeping men silent, therefore helping male mental health become the national discussion point it is today.

My work experience involved a mix of office assistant tasks and writing articles for the *CALMzine* magazine, about anything from the testicular cancer scare I'd had as a teenager to a love letter to Stephen Fry. One part of the job was also going through the news each day and finding articles about male suicide and seeing how they'd been covered and reported. Whilst I was there, it was widely reported that Stephen Fry, national comedy treasure, patron of Mind and a prolific mental health campaigner, had attempted to take his own life a few months previously. Some of the media had reported this quite irresponsibly and Rachel began telling me some of the reasons why.

The representation of suicide in popular media has long been affected by the stigma of suicide having once been an illegal act. In 1961, under the UK's Suicide Act, suicide was decriminalised, meaning those who made failed attempts would not be prosecuted. Over half a century later, however, our press still continue to use the verb 'commit' in our national newspapers to describe the act of someone taking their own life. Rachel described how this bolsters the connotations that suicide is a selfish act. That the word 'commit' helps continue a historic stigma of blame and shame on vulnerable people who end their life. She told me how the language of suicide reporting can also be incredibly dangerous. Many academics and researchers have accused Western media outlets in particular of taking risks with their coverage of suicidal incidents, with numerous studies showing conclusive evidence of negative, inappropriate and irresponsible coverage of suicide leading to 'copycat suicides' and influencing suicidal ideation, a term for someone thinking about ending their own life, amongst vulnerable readers.

Charities like CALM and the Samaritans work with media ethics regulators to monitor reporting and give guidance to journalists on best practice, and that's why CALM wanted me to log how male suicides were being reported whilst I was doing this internship.

All of a sudden, this whole issue felt like such an important and interesting topic for my dissertation. I was both passionate about this idea and intrigued. I wanted to look at the way our newspapers sensationalise suicide in order to sell copies, and how that can have a devastatingly tragic effect on readers and the loved ones of those involved.

One personal reason I had for choosing this topic was hearing what had happened to Cecilia after Leo's suicide. His death was reported by the local press in Brighton, including the method of his suicide, which was a relatively rare one, and reporters had bothered both her and her dad for more details when they were in the deepest pits of their grief. It was completely inappropriate and nobody could actually do anything to stop it, except ignore the press and hope they went away.

So I got in touch with the Samaritans who regularly hand out suicide reporting guidelines to media outlets and freelance journalists. I've picked out a couple that I want you guys to read, because it's also important that, in conversations we have with potentially vulnerable friends or loved ones, we stick to these. I believe they should be guidelines for all of society when talking about suicide.

SAMARITANS MEDIA GUIDELINES

Details of suicide methods have been shown to prompt vulnerable individuals to imitate suicidal behaviour. With this in mind, Samaritans recommends:

- Avoid giving too much detail. Care should be taken when giving any detail of a suicide method.
- Avoid any mention of the method in headlines, as this inadvertently promotes and perpetuates common methods of suicide.

- Take extra care when reporting the facts of cases where an unusual or previously unknown method has been used. Incidences of people using unusual or new methods of suicide have been known to increase rapidly after being reported widely. Reporting may also drive people to the internet to search for more information about these methods.
- Remember that there is a risk of imitational behaviour due to 'over-identification'. Vulnerable individuals may identify with a person who has died, or with the circumstances in which a person took their own life. For example, combining references to life circumstances, debt problems, job loss AND descriptions of an easy-to-imitate suicide method in the same report could put at greater risk people who are vulnerable as a result of financial stress.

And so these guidelines in particular became the basis for my dissertation. I wanted to analyse three incidents of suicide that were reported in our national newspapers and see whether the journalists writing the story or their editors listened to these ethics or disregarded them to sensationalise and sell papers.

final year of uni

September 2013–March 2014

My final year of university was much like my second, except Lewis, Brendan and I did knuckle down a bit more. And by 'knuckling down', I mean that instead of getting drunk every other day in the pub, we did it on the sofa in Lewis's room, all of us with our laptops open to feign the act of doing work while simultaneously drinking.

Brendan and I would each take it in turns to do the rounds of our local supermarkets, sending photos of reduced food with yellow discount stickers to one another on a daily basis. One day I'd be grabbing 37p tuna sandwiches, the next day Brendan would come home with an M&S charcuterie board reduced from £25 down to £3.99. This meant we were eating luxury cured meats and cheeses for a whole week whilst writing our dissertations.

We fell into a routine of staying up late into the night and working. Having just lost a friend to suicide, Brendan particularly noticed all my academic research texts about suicide prevention laying around the flat. He'd say things like, 'Jack, you know what your *Mastermind* specialist subject should be?'

'Er, dunno, what should it be, Brendan?'

'Well, if M.I.A.'s discography isn't available, then it should be suicide, because you have twenty-eight books about it taking over the kitchen table!'

I felt bad as, back then, I hadn't actually been directly affected by suicide, but I knew, deep down, Brendan was quite proud I'd picked that topic.

As we would sit together working on our dissertations until 3am, we'd sometimes stretch our legs and head over to the trusty 24-hour Nisa Local down the road for late-night snacks. The shop was open so infinitely that it didn't even have a door!

'What if it's snowing?' I'd say to Khalid behind the counter, who would just smile and nod that they still didn't need one.

On these 3am visits I would often bump into two particular celebrities: Gail Porter and Bill Nighy, the pair of them also naughty late-night Nisa regulars. We would silently nod to each other, like, 'Yes, Gail, it is 3am, but I want some Milky Way Magic Stars and nothing's gonna stop me!'

Meanwhile, Olly had left university and was working at a relatively good magazine in Soho. We still chatted every now and then. One time he called me out of the blue, dripping with excitement that he'd written his first proper article about how the new Pope loved the gays.

'Jack, mate, this new Pope, he loves the gays!'

'Thank you for telling me this, Olly, but I don't think it fully makes up for all the other shit the previous popes have been peddling!'

Sometimes I'd meet Olly once he'd finished work and we would go to his favourite pub. In February 2014 he told me that he was finding everything quite tough. I think a lot of graduates struggle that first year, when they find themselves thrown in the deep end of professional employment without both the structure and freedom of university, or the relative comfort of a Student Finance England safety net. But that day I could really tell that his mood had changed. His temperament since leaving university had seemed duller – like he'd lost a bit of his colour. He'd struggled finding work placements and then to find his feet in his job, and was still feeling quite low. He just wasn't wearing himself very well, if that makes sense. Instead, life was wearing him.

I tried to counsel him around this time, and invited him to the odd comedy night I'd started doing in an attempt to cheer him up. I'd decided to move away from poetry and I'd signed up to a stand-up course at Soho Theatre. I tried out some very ropey stand-up material at some local pub comedy nights, which he would gently chuckle along to.

And whilst he was happy for me, I could still sense he was really down. Olly had a more complex mental illness than any of my experiences with anxiety and depression. From what I gather, he had been misdiagnosed psychiatrically in the past – something that happens quite frequently in the realm of mental illnesses. He was told he was bipolar, told he had borderline personality disorder, was moved from one medication to another medication – anti-psychotics, mood-stabilisers, anti-depressants, the lot. At the time he never fully told me the extent of what was happening or how it was affecting him. I don't know the full details so I don't want to speculate any further, but I do know that we were very frank and honest with each other about our emotions and the times we were struggling with feeling shit.

Olly asked me about how my third year was going and I told him about my dissertation on suicide-reporting media ethics. He thought it was great and I vaguely remember him saying something along the lines of 'The media can be such cunts.' Olly and I regularly talked at great length about how the media can fuck us up. About how societal depictions of class, sexuality, mental health – all of them can perpetuate stereotypes which just damage the most vulnerable.

At the time, there was a television series on Channel 4 called *Benefits Street*, which had kicked up quite a fuss in the media, with many branding it controversial poverty porn – a reality show disguised as a documentary that could be deemed by some to exploit the impoverished subjects featured in each episode. One of these was a woman called 'White Dee', who spoke about being diagnosed with bipolar and whom a lot of the tabloid press attacked, claiming her mental illness was just a sob story.

Olly defended the show and we had a bit of a tense back and forth over our opinions. But I remember him passionately saying that he thought any exposure of the clusterfuck that was Britain's mental health crisis was an important thing to see, and that watching how society struggles to support working-class people was something others should watch.

Olly, being six years older than me, with different life experiences, taught me a lot about why people need ambition, how it helped him to get out of a hole in his life, and why people need to fight those background limitations placed on them.

At the time we were having these chats, in early 2014, we were going into the last year of an austerity-led coalition government that had devastated mental health services. Child and adolescent mental health services, or CAMHS, had been scaled back in a lot of areas; in some, they'd been completely decimated – destroyed by cuts, staff losses and lack of provision for emergency care to get to the most vulnerable young people in the most vulnerable areas.

Volunteering at CALM around this time had made me realise that, whilst more people were becoming aware of CALM as a campaign to help young men, this had resulted in more demand for help. People were opening up more about mental health issues, depression and anxiety, because there was greater coverage of awareness raising campaigns to get people to open up.

But who to? As the demand grew and the rate of male suicide remained disproportionally high, mental health services began experiencing ever growing waiting lists. I also started to notice around this time that mental health was beginning to be used by certain companies and organisations, because of its mass appeal, to tap into people's very real personal struggles. Some of these companies, though not all, were starting to manipulate those struggles I felt, as part of an 'awareness conversation', which was very little about raising awareness of how better to help people and more about raising awareness of their own brand. These companies very quickly found they were benefitting from the mental health conversation by appearing caring and like they were fighting stigma by encouraging people to talk, but actually doing very little to stop the cuts to services that were actually saving people's lives.

The more crucial issue back then was that we didn't and still today do not need everyone to engage in just talking about talking. What we need is talking then *action*, and for those waiting lists and services to be better funded, repaired and made available for people when they really need it. CALM was one charity out of many trying to help people when our government were not doing enough.

And on that night in the pub, as me and Olly finished our pints, he remarked that he was thinking of moving back home to the coast. I told him to stick at his job and that it was just a blip. A few months later, he left London.

broke with expensive taste

March–May 2014

It's quite embarrassing that my main memories of my third year don't evoke tales of studious discipline or creative discovery; they do, however, involve the procurement of cheap, out-of-date food. Close to my university's 24-hour library, where me and Brendan would occasionally work, was a branch of the soup and sushi franchise Itsu. Each day, half an hour before they close at 21.00, Itsu outlets reduce all their food by 50 per cent. Some of you may have been competitors in an Itsu half-price sale, but the half-price sale in *this particular* branch on London's Baker Street was a highly competitive, Black-Friday-esque scramble that was dangerous to enter into. At 20.25 each day, you could witness great men fall before the last teriyaki salmon rice box, or two women in digital marketing row over a pot of edamame pods or, sadly, watch an old lady have her spine crushed in a stampede for cheap fresh-fruit smoothies.

To avoid these horrors, Brendan and I developed a strategy that enabled us to be ready and prepared for 20.30, when all that fresh food would be slashed in price. We took the timings of this incredibly seriously, calculating that if we left the library at 20.07 at the very latest, we could get to Itsu for 20.19 and start grabbing the grub we wanted, then sit on a stool close to the tills, ready to bag a discount and be back to work by 20.45. It was a military operation, which we conducted with absolute precision. Then we would take up whole swathes of library desk space, spreading out a buffet of freshly-made-that-morning sushi that was slowly rotting.

Around this time one of my favourite rappers, Azealia Banks, released her long-awaited debut album, *Broke With Expensive Taste*, and that very much became my personal brand for a short time – how to live a bouji life whilst being super skint.

Halfway through my dissertation, in March 2014, I got a phone call from my cousin Amy, telling me to come home. My Uncle Saff had had a heart attack and died very suddenly. He was sixty-four. It was the first major loss we'd experienced since my dad. Uncle Saff was on my mum's side of the family, and he was just one of the kindest, most harmless men you could ever hope to meet. He was a haulage skip driver, who'd spend eight hours a day in a massive vehicle which he'd toot the horn of ridiculously loudly every Friday when he saw me walking home from school.

After a couple days grieving at Mum's, I returned to our flat to find Brendan making us a huge breakfast spread of pancakes, bacon and maple syrup, to cheer me up. It remains one of the sweetest gestures anyone's ever done for me, because none of the food was reduced. He'd bought it all full price!

I got back to university and my journalism lecturer Patrick said he would help me with anything I needed, pushing back some deadlines on other projects so I could just knuckle down with the mammoth dissertation I had tangled myself in. I found it too tough to even process that Saff was gone, and so I did the unhealthy but perhaps necessary thing of pushing it to the back of my mind and powering on. The deadline day was in sight!

how to tell work or uni that you need time off

Mental health in the workplace/place of education is a crucial topic that I hope people are starting to take more seriously. I read a heartbreaking *VICE* article at the end of 2019 by a brilliant writer, Hannah Ewens, about the high rates of suicide at just one higher education establishment – Bristol University. She wrote: 'In the 18 months between October of 2016 and April of 2018, 11 Bristol University students died by suspected suicide. In the year-and-a-half since, that number has risen to at least 13.'

Students struggling with poor mental health around the country has become a real crisis. Likewise, workplaces have had to tackle similar issues regarding employee stress and the effects of workloads on people's daily wellbeing. With all this in mind, I think it's very important to speak up and tell your lecturers/your bosses. If you or someone you're worried about has an HR team at work, then obviously there may be internal processes, but do not ever feel scared to open up and ask for help.

You'd also be surprised at how much people want to help. There are now more and more new schemes popping up, like Mental Health First Aid in the workplace, where a designated person in an organisation is sent off for training in giving assistance to employees who run into mental health difficulties. A lot of universities will also have protocols in place, like 'mitigating circumstances', to help you during your studies. Make sure you or someone you're worried about finds out what support is available for your campus or workplace.

I would also say that, currently, many universities are prioritising putting more funding and time into mental health services. If they are not, then try to use the student union of that campus to campaign for those changes. It really is so important and I believe that, gradually, we are getting on a better track.

deadline day

May 2014

The night before handing my dissertation in, I went into a full-on meltdown and pulled an all-nighter. I wore my slippers in the library and purchased a dangerous pack of six Monster Red energy drinks. If there's a mental wellbeing tip I want to emphasise in this book it's NEVER BUY THAT MANY ENERGY DRINKS.

Lily sat next to me, rushing her appendix, next to her was Tom, who worked in the North London Tavern and wrote his whole thesis in ten hours. He later got a high 2:1 and I honestly don't understand how he did it. Night turned into the next morning and by 11am I thought I was finally done.

Olly came up to university that day and he wanted to hand in my dissertation with me. Sitting in the library, he read through bits and he was just acting quite weird, jittery almost. I asked him what was wrong and he wouldn't say, and because I was in such a rush I didn't have time to probe him any further.

My dissertation was titled: 'A study into the ethics of UK press coverage on suicide.'

This is the abstract from my study:

The purpose of this study was to investigate the ethical practices of newspaper reports on suicide, analysing whether or not newspapers adhere to media guidelines and editorial ethics codes on responsible reporting.

The study examined three national newspapers, conducting an interpretative content analysis to conclude how suicide is represented and which specific media guidelines are adhered to.

The study recommends that improvements need to be made in terms of ethical guideline adherence and sensitive reporting from both tabloid and broadsheet titles.

The study also suggests that editors and journalists need to be held accountable for when their work mentions the method of someone's suicide, especially when suicide is a prevalent issue in vulnerable groups of society, such as young people and those suffering with mental health issues.

Once I'd finished typing up the last bits, Olly suggested we had lunch so I could re-read my conclusion before handing it in.

We sat in the uni canteen and very soon I could tell he wasn't himself. He started telling me how the doctors had put him on new medication again and that he couldn't sleep properly. He kept on jittering, twitching, his eyes seemed really tired yet intense. This was making me feel very anxious, because he was so manic. Two common side effects of anti-psychotic medication are having abnormal movements of the face or body and difficulty concentrating in conversations. Back then, I didn't know that. This deadline day was such a huge deal for me, essentially finishing my three years of study, yet a part of me felt that Olly had come along and been quite demanding and erratic, and I didn't understand why.

We found out over lunch that neither of us had slept properly in days. I had been awake for around 32 hours. For some reason, we chose chicken madras off the menu. As we sat there, I tried my hardest to listen to him whilst being desperately tired and just wanting to hand in the whole dissertation and go to bed. Then, after two or three mouthfuls, all of a sudden I started having choking-like symptoms. I just couldn't swallow anything and soon enough I descended into panic.

Now, I'm not sure if you've ever tried to eat a chicken madras after not having slept for 32 hours but – it doesn't work. As I panicked, Olly just sat there, doing nothing. I staggered across to try to get a bottle of water, but the till woman actually said '£1.20' and I couldn't tell her 'I need water I think I'm choking', because ... I was choking! Someone passed me an Evian and a chunk of chicken flew out of my mouth, as two first-year students checked that I was OK. I'd gone bright red and was sweating buckets. But throughout the whole thing Olly had continued to just sit there, head down in his plate, twitching and eating his madras. Once I'd calmed down, I sat back at the table and I saw that Olly had eaten most of my madras too.

And that's when I knew something was wrong with him. There was something about his behaviour that was so manic, it was scary almost. I think he thought I'd just upped and left and was completely oblivious as to why I'd gotten up in the first place.

We headed back to the library. I printed, bound and handed in my dissertation and then went to the bar to cheers! But after not sleeping for 35 hours, by this point I was so exhausted I couldn't be cheerful. I realised that I'd been powering on since Uncle Saff died, working every night to avoid catching up with my emotions, and then all of a sudden, it was done.

That night I hugged Olly goodbye and he said he might need to stay with me for a couple of nights the following week. I told him to message me and we could sort something. The next day I sent him a text, checking in on him. He didn't text back and I was worried I'd annoyed him. I didn't fully understand what he was going through.

my nan, Sicely

June 2014

After Dad died, the thing I longed for the most was to hear his voice. I so badly missed his bizarre little sayings and the way he'd recount the stories that had come from the back of his black cab that day. And so I started recording his mum (my nan), speaking all about her life into a Dictaphone.

This started off as just something I wanted to do, so that one day, when she died, I could still listen to her. I would always have something concrete to reminisce over, which for me felt more evocative than a photograph. We did these little recording sessions around two or three times a year, perhaps on Mother's Day or Father's Day after dinner, when Nan was relaxed and I could ask her all about her life before me.

Whilst I was finishing up my studies, I wanted to make use of the fact that being at a media campus meant I could hire out a wealth of equipment for free to make stuff, and so I decided to get out a camera and some microphones and start trying to shoot a personal documentary about grief. Something factual combining all the stories from my poems and all the thoughts I had on how awkward Britain is about death. Brendan agreed to help me.

The first person I wanted to interview on camera was Nan. She was quite poorly at the time and kept suffering with extreme stomach pains, but she sweetly agreed that me and Brendan could come round hers to film us having lunch on Father's Day and us talking all about my dad, the idea being that this would give us a main interview to act as the spine of a documentary about different generations dealing with bereavement, capturing a teenage perspective alongside that of an elderly person.

So, on the middle Sunday of June 2014, me and Brendan travelled up to her council flat in Uxbridge and had a bizarre buffet with her and my grandad of pretty much anything which was in the freezer that Nan wanted to get rid of.

Sadly, by this time, my grandad's dementia was quite advanced and we decided he wasn't the best person to interview. Talking about my dad was something he couldn't do, not even to Nan. Despite being physically ill herself, Nan was essentially his carer, which was an additional pressure on her, but she felt it was important to speak about Dad and grief.

So, after we'd had food, Nan and me sat at her kitchen table and spoke all about my dad as a little boy, about him becoming a father, his career in mechanics, his romance with my mum and then finally his death. We chatted about what it was like for her to lose a child and how that's such a taboo, uncomfortable topic. And my nan, in her honest, frank way, gave such beautiful testimonials of my dad's life and wise musings on loss, love and the power of carrying on against the odds. Some moments were funny and touching whilst others were heartbreakingly sad. She spoke about how my grandad sometimes asked her where my dad was, questioning her on why he hadn't visited recently. And then she had to tell him, 'He's gone. Laurence is gone', and relive that moment all over again. It was something I hadn't realised that she had had to cope with.

She explained that whilst friends of hers would be fine talking about an elderly friend from bingo who'd passed away, she felt too awkward to ever talk about her own son. And she so desperately wanted to remember him, talk about him and celebrate his life.

At one point in the interview my grandad popped in to sweetly enquire whether Nan wanted to watch *Emmerdale*, and she was comically short tempered with him – 'Oh bugger off, John, it's 4.30! *Emmerdale* ain't on till 7!'

And there were all these funny moments of her in real life as an eighty-five-year-old woman, who was a mother to a child she'd lost, a wife to a partner who was severely losing his faculties, and a grandmother to me, who just wanted for her to escape and bake apple pies and not have the weight of the world on her shoulders.

In last scene we filmed, I am wrapping up my questions and she asks me if I want any apple pie. I say, 'Oh yes, please, do you have any double cream?'

And she turns round and says, 'No, darl, I've only got single but I could give you double the amount?'

And with that final frame, tracking in on a cheeky grin from her, we see me give her a kiss on the cheek and then Brendan shouting cut.

In the pit of my stomach, when watching back the edit, I had an inkling that this one film was going to be the thing I threw myself into making. That it was going to be something special.

graduation and prank calls

July–October 2014

My graduation ceremony was at the Royal Festival Hall in July, on the hottest day of the year – and yes, your boy Jack got a first! Sadly I wasn't smart enough to pre-book my cap and gown, so muggins here had to arrive at 7.30am to sort it out. Me and Lewis went together, got into our graduation attire by 8.30, and then waited outside the nearest pub for it to open and so we could get pissed up in the sunshine.

By the time the graduation ceremony started at 2pm, I was absolutely wasted. Truly, truly shitfaced. A video my brother took of me receiving my scroll on stage shows me wobbling up some steps, shaking the wrong person's hand and then running across the Royal Festival Hall stage into five rows of lecturers sat on the stage, clasping my lecturer Patrick's shoulder to hug him for getting me through it all. I completely disrupted the alphabetical order of graduation and then was taken off to sober up outside. It was wonderful.

That same month, Rachel from CALM asked if I would deputy edit the *CALMzine* with her, which I was over the moon about, and then a mini dream of mine came true and I got offered a paid part-time job working on Radio 1's *The Surgery*, partly because of all my experience working for CALM and speaking to young people. *The Surgery* was a long-running weekly call-in show for teenage listeners, where they could ring up about a whole host of issues affecting them, with episodes on everything from exam stress to STIs.

When someone called to speak on-air to the lead presenter and a studio doctor, I would be that first person they'd get through to. My job was to safeguard any younger people ringing in and offer them helplines and advice, whilst also finding good editorial stories and questions for the presenters to answer live on air with the caller patched into the studio. I had to prepare the caller, rehearsing with them how they could concisely introduce their problem on air in less than 30 seconds, while making sure that the young person on the other end of the line actually felt confident enough to speak on air and wasn't going to erupt into floods of tears, and also that it wasn't a prank.

During my time in this job, only twice did I patch through someone who, as soon as the presenter said, 'Hey there, what's your problem?' shouted in response: 'FUCK ME IN THE PUSSY!' before putting down the phone and hanging up. Apparently, the infrequency of this happening on my watch meant I was very good at detecting potential prank callers. I think that's because, as someone who used to prank call my nan all the time as a child, I inherently recognise the signals of a true prankster! If anyone giggled during their preliminary phone chat with me, or if I heard anyone chuckling or whispering in the background, I would refuse to put them on air and just fob them off with the BBC Action line, at which point they'd just scream 'FUCK ME IN THE PUSSY' at me, rather than the whole Radio 1 audience. I was very proud of this achievement.

Everything was going very well, but I still hadn't heard much from Olly. Apart from the odd text here and there, he'd generally vanished, being vague with plans to meet up, meaning we never did. And I was so busy doing comedy gigs and trying out stand-up sets that I just didn't have time to chase him up.

I'd met a comedian called Camille who was part of a comedy sketch group called Birthday Girls. We'd done some gigs together, got pissed at some parties and eventually realised we got on rather well. She'd broken up with her fella and was looking for somewhere in London to live; meanwhile I'd moved out of my uni flat and was living back at my mum's and still keeping my sexuality a secret. I was getting quite desperate to move out and so Camille and I came up with a plan.

Camille was a property guardian, and while the waiting lists were ridiculously long, if Camille was to leave the current guardianship she was in with her ex, she could move into another property and me being her friend would bump me up the list. They clocked that friends who live together, stay together, and the longer you stay, the more you pay.

So this is exactly what happened. However, the nature of guardianships is that you turn up to view a property and then you've got to scramble to reserve rooms if you like it, making the decision and signing the contracts almost immediately. (This goes against everything I said in the advice guide about how best to know who to live with, because you don't really get a choice.)

We went to look round an ex-care home in Willesden Green, which we saw for about six minutes before bagsying two rooms for £350 per month including bills. Then we realised it was an absolute dive. It felt haunted; you could tell a helluva lotta old people had died there.

After one week, Camille ran into my room one night and said, 'Jack, my tits have been bitten to shit. Have yours?'

'Er, yes, I *have* been a bit itchy.'

The place was riddled with bed bugs.

After seven days of co-habitation, we were again without somewhere to live. Camille was re-housed in an amazing guardianship in Soho and I was put on a priority list, though I had to move back in with my mum, tail firmly between my legs.

At the time I was still hosting Bang Said the Gun and one day a writer called Nathan Penlington came and performed. He had created his own show based on the 'Choose Your Own Adventure' books, where he'd filmed all the possible outcomes of trying to track down a man in real life whose diary he'd found when it fell out of a 'Choose Your Own Adventure' book that Nathan purchased on eBay. Watching him in this show, cutting between video and storytelling, was gripping. The audience had keypads and would vote for different things to happen, like in the books – or, for millennials, like in *Black Mirror: Bandersnatch*! It was like a live comedy documentary and I became obsessed with trying to blend comedy and documentary together in a live show.

I met a woman called Sarah at a funding organisation called Arts Council England who said I could apply for a grant to turn my stories and films about grief into a similar live project to Nathan's. I started to think that, rather than trying to make a documentary film and bankrupting myself in the process, I would apply for an Arts Council grant to create a live comedy-theatre show, co-written with my nan and combining the interviews I'd filmed with her on Father's Day, with me performing some comedy stories about grief.

I asked Nan if she'd be up for it and she said she was just feeling too ill to do anything live on stage or that involved coming into London, but that she was very happy for me to chop up our interview and contribute to stories around each one. That was more than enough for me to play with, so I applied for a grant and thankfully got the cash!

I called Nan to tell her and she said, 'Brilliant! So where will you be doing this live show?'

'Er, I dunno, probably just a small arts centre to start with.'

And she sighed and said, 'Oh, I thought you'd be talking like the Palladium or something. Quite a few comedians do shows there nowadays.'

'No, Nan. I'm thinking more a room above a pub where I'd be lucky if people even stopped talking to notice a show was going on.'

Nan needed to be a bit more impressed.

good grief

November 2014

Do you remember Hayley Cropper from *Coronation Street*? She was married to good old Roy who ran the café and she was the first transgender character in a British soap opera, until she sadly died in 2014. For her funeral, Hayley shuffled off this mortal coil in a floral-patterned eco-friendly cardboard coffin, in an episode watched by nearly 8 million people, who tuned in to say goodbye to the iconic HC. Ten months after her funeral, this prop coffin was donated to me by the Natural Death Centre and I filled it up with bags of Wotsits, custard creams, Monster Munch and a Coca-Cola bottle that said 'Share a Coke with Dad', which I'd Sharpie'd the word 'Dead' on to. This prop became the centrepiece for my very first show, *Good Grief*.

I did what's called a 'research and development' week of the show at the Roundhouse in Camden, trying out some funny stories I'd written on loss alongside the video interviews of my nan.

Audience members would walk in and straight away have to drop off some bereavement comfort food into the coffin, while I stood behind it and thanked them for their contribution and then off they would go to take their seats. It was a darkly comic send-up of the British etiquette of grief. Throughout the show, I would get food out of the coffin and feed the audience slices of buttered Soreen, just like my dad brought me when he told me he had cancer. Then I would give them custard cream biscuits so they could taste what weeks of visiting family during grief can often feel like. I even got one audience member each show to put my dad's phone number into their phone contacts and promise to never delete it so they could feel that moment when you're scrolling through and see the digits of someone you can no longer call.

I told the story about how I used to use my school's Get Out of Class card to bunk off lessons and get sympathy from teachers, and then I gave out to the audience adult versions of these cards, called Get Out of Shit Event – or GOOSE – cards. They were little business cards with a photo of me and my dad on one side and the other side said ...

Please excuse 'insert name; from your show/party/ situation. They may feel down/upset/tired of you, and require some alone time with their thoughts/biscuit tin/ copy of the Radio Times'
Signed, Jack Rooke | Expires – NEVER!

The show was a mix of silly spontaneous comedy and more theatrical moments of pathos that I thought would help capture the whole world of bereavement. From the audience feedback, I found out that what people loved the most was when we talked about pranking one another – like how my nan used to pretend she'd left a slice of homemade cake for me in the fridge on a plate under a bowl, and then I'd lift it up and there'd just be some cut-up carrot sticks with a note saying 'GOTCHA, FATTY'. (Before any millennials call my nan out for fat shaming me, please just know that she fed me cake almost every waking hour I spent with her, so she actually did love me podgy.)

The audience feedback also said that they loved us talking about how we manipulated our grief and others' sympathy to get what we wanted out of people! And so I re-wrote bits of the script as the research week went on, calling Nan to check in with her and trying to get the perfect balance of stories: sadness mixed with fun moments mixed with mischief and all tied up with pathos to boot!

The very last scene of this draft of *Good Grief* was everyone's favourite: this was that last bit of video of me and Nan joking about in her kitchen and eating apple pie. Every audience that week cried at that moment and, without sounding too manipulative, I just knew by the end of these work-in-progress shows that mine and Nan's show was on to something. In my mind the next step was trying to convince a big venue at the Edinburgh Fringe to take a chance on me as a relatively unknown act and give me a slot for the festival. This became the plan!

And then, the morning after that week of initial performances, my nan went into hospital.

She'd been ill for quite a few months, too ill to even come and watch me perform the show, and she was in such a lot of pain that the hospital said they'd look after her for a bit. Meanwhile, my grandad was put in a temporary care home to give my nan some respite.

And that same Saturday morning, a producer who had seen the show the night before booked me to perform a 15-minute snippet of it the following Saturday at the Trafalgar Studios in the West End, as part of a showcase night that Meera Syal was hosting. I was ridiculously excited – the fact I was going to do any of it in the West End before it had even been on in a fringe theatre felt like another good sign that this show could do well.

I spent all that week rehearsing this 15-minute set, refining it, making it perfect. And then, four days later, on the Wednesday before the gig, the doctors found that my nan had a tumour blocking her bowel. They said that they wanted her to give full permission to operate and remove it as soon as possible, but there were potential ramifications if they couldn't fully remove it. This growth was what was causing her such constant pain.

Me and my mum spoke to her on the phone and Nan said two words I'd never heard her say before.

'I'm scared.'

And the truth was, we were scared too. But she'd been getting so increasingly unwell and frail in the last few years that we told her we thought she should agree to the operation. The worst-case scenario was that she'd need part of her bowel removed and a colostomy bag fitted and we told her we'd support her whatever happened.

Then I grabbed the phone and said, 'Nan, you've got to do this, OK? I promise it'll be fine. And now enough about you, I'm doing our show in the West End on Saturday with Meera Syal!'

Nan laughed and said, 'Ooh, you're getting closer to the Palladium then?'

'Yes, maybe one day.'

She chirped up and ended our phone call with, 'Well here's me giving you a big kiss, well done.'

The next day she had the operation and they successfully removed the growth.

Saturday came and I did the gig with Meera Syal. Not sure if I mentioned it, but it was in THE WEST END! And afterwards I was on cloud nine. It was maybe at that point one of the best gigs I'd ever done.

The day after, my dad's brother, Uncle Clive, called us after visiting Nan at the hospital.

He said, with his voice cracking in between each word, 'The doctors reckon she's got one to two weeks left. Her organs are failing and she's not gonna pull through.'

I demanded Mum take me to the hospital that very minute and she said, 'No, don't be silly, we'll go up and see her tomorrow.'

But this huge paranoia came over me and I just ran upstairs, got dressed, put on my dad's watch and grabbed my nan a Get Out of Shit Event card. She'd wanted to see them the week before, and I wanted her to see that, on the other side of this card, was a picture of me and my dad – the exact same photo she kept in her purse.

When we got to the ICU, Mum and Uncle Clive went in to see Nan first. After 20 minutes or so, they came back and my mum held my shoulders and said, 'Don't be scared. She's not really with it. She's not speaking as she's hooked up to air.'

And I was shaking. I was really, really shaking.

I walked into the ICU, went up to her bed, pulled back the curtain and there she was – lying on her back, hooked up to machines and fighting. She wasn't able to speak as the morphine dose she was on was so high, but they informed me she could hear what I was saying. The whole thing felt very similar to my dad.

And then, as I stepped into the bay she was in, all of a sudden I just stopped shaking. I became very, very calm. I sat next to her and stroked her hand, telling her I was there. By this point, the doctor had told my Uncle Clive he thought she had three or four days left, but the first thought that came into my mind was, 'I hope it's less.' In that moment, I just wanted for her to go.

But even on her deathbed I couldn't resist just chatting to her like normal.

'Nan, I did that gig last night with Meera Syal in the West End. And I did the show last week, and everyone who saw you, loved you. Everyone loves you!'

I gave her a big kiss well done and put one of the little Get Out of Shit Event cards with me and Dad on it next to her bed.

Good grief

After about 40 minutes, I left to go sit in the waiting room for a break. Mum followed and we went to get a Costa Express coffee, as if things weren't depressing enough! And as we came back into the corridor of the ICU, my uncle came up to us and said, 'She's gone.'

This person who I had been speaking to all month, whose voice I'd just spent a week editing in every video for the show, was suddenly gone. I couldn't believe it.

We all just hugged for what felt like the longest 15 seconds of my life and then the doctor poked his head around the door and said, 'Sorry um ... she's not actually passed. She's still breathing if you wanna ... '

I interrupted with the loudest nervous laugh of my entire life.

We rushed to return to her bed and, as I sat there, I thought, 'Ahh, she's pranked me! She's got me! She got me one last time. She's bloody won!!'

Another few minutes passed until my nan went to sleep and didn't wake up.

And it was one of the funniest, most beautiful things I had ever seen.

I had to change the end of the show after she'd passed. This story of the West End gig and her prank death became the eventual ending. I would let the audience believe she was alive for 55 minutes and that we were talking only about my dad's passing, and then I'd tell that story. It turned Good Grief from a fairly good comedy show in the first draft into something that would have whole audiences in floods of laughter and tears.

To finish off, I played the apple pie video of her telling me she could give me double the amount of single cream as she winked to camera, all whilst I lifted out a freshly baked apple pie on a gold tray from the coffin, put it on my lap, cut out one slice and rested it on the coffin for Nan. I then poured two pots of single cream all over the other 85 per cent of the pie, all to myself, and, just as I took a huge bite, the lights would black out.

Mine and Nan's show was done.

coffin boy

January 2015

I eventually got offered a place in a property guardianship, an office block above a car garage near Hampstead Heath. There were fifteen of us and it was pretty much like uni halls for adults, except everyone could just smoke weed inside because no one really made the rules in guardianships. They were relatively lawless places unless the guardianship company or landlord made a random check on your property, in which case everyone would rush to do a Mary Poppins-esque tidy up, even if they were high on MKat.

You'd only get a warning if they caught you being 'naughty', which for most people was never, and for me it was always fine because I never did any drugs stronger than paracetamol whilst I was there. Just one guy called David always got caught, and he'd literally be snorting coke off any available surface he could find at any given moment. I'd go in the kitchen and I'd see him in a corner racking up lines. One time I had to tell him off, shouting, 'You are literally snorting coke off my packet of fucking Uncle Ben's microwave rice! I'm about to heat that up!' David was a nice lad at heart and I bloody well hope he's all right now, whatever he's up to.

When I first arrived with all my stuff, everyone came and greeted me to say hello, but I soon realised the housemate situation changed every few weeks, so who I met at the start would evolve on a regular basis. As there were always new people moving in and out, making good first impressions counted in the world of guardianships – make a bad first impression and you could expect to get the worst choice of cupboard in the kitchen and be left out of any group picnics on the heath.

When I arrived, I walked in holding a six-foot-three floral cardboard coffin, so all the sane people in the guardianship avoided me, nicknaming me 'Coffin Boy', while all the weirdos in the guardianship absolutely loved me, and also nicknamed me 'Coffin Boy'. Basically, my whole identity was boiled down to 'boy with coffin', which is a distinctive first impression to make, and I'd recommend anyone looking to join a property guardianship scheme find a coffin to accompany them.

Once I told everyone what the coffin was for, they all started coming to see preview performances of my show and asking if they could pinch a bag of Monster Munch. Everyone was much more supportive when they realised the coffin was 'for art'.

My room was situated in between those of a Nordic fitness addict, an events girl, a stoner skateboarder and a part-time webcam girl, called Daisy. The walls were office walls, so they were almost paper thin, and some nights I could hear Daisy fake-orgasming for the odd £75 here and there, minus commission. She was really, really lovely.

Daisy would let me come into her room and dick about after work, order in twenty chicken wings and try on all her fancy silk scarfs as if I were Bridget Jones in a boat with Daniel Cleaver on their dirty hotel weekend. Daisy would tell me all about her exciting sex life, from shagging her boss on a glass office boardroom table after work to having a girl go down on her for 45 minutes straight. It was a bit like living next to a non-famous, bisexual Amy Schumer.

Because my room was an ex-office, it had horrible strip lighting, so instead I sourced twenty mix-and-match lamps with a whole 400m Olympic running track of fairy lights going around the walls. My window looked out on the overground line, where other housemates would occasionally throw water bombs at all the trendy millennials going swimming in the Hampstead ponds, just so they could put it on Instagram.

The week I moved in, me and Lewis went to visit our friend and Olly's ex-housemate, Claire, in her property guardianship, a car park building right around the corner in Chalk Farm, directly opposite the Roundhouse where I'd been performing. It was the first time I'd spoken about Olly for months, as we still hadn't met up. I just presumed that it was because of life getting in the way. It's quite common when everyone graduates from university and your lives go in different directions.

Claire and I laughed about how he would be too much of a princess to live in a guardianship and she told me to just send him a text telling him that she and I now lived round the corner from each other again, so he should come up and see us.

I said, 'I think he'll be annoyed with me that we haven't spoken in ages.'

And Claire looked at me, with little time for my paranoia, and said, 'No he won't, just text him, you lazy cow.'

The following week, me and Olly spoke on the phone on what would have been my dad's sixty-second birthday. We had a good hour-long catch-up chat, beginning with how we both had jip with our radiators and then how we'd both been having a bit of a bad time. I told him all about my nan's passing and he told me that he'd been feeling quite up and down recently but was hoping to go to Japan soon to see his dad and perhaps do some teaching out there. I thought this was a brilliant idea.

We had a laugh and a reminisce about the uni days. He said how he'd been living in Chichester full-time with some flatmates and working at Clarks shoe shop to get in some money. At the time, I was applying to become a primary school teaching assistant with a teaching agency, trying to get any cash I could to help me fund taking *Good Grief* to Edinburgh.

And at the end of this catch-up call, I remember Olly telling me to keep my chin up, that 'it'll happen'. We ended the call with him making plans to come up and see me and Claire at some point before Easter and me promising I'd come down to the seaside in spring. And I would like to believe that they were genuine plans. Plans that Olly meant to keep. But sadly neither of those things ever happened.

the pitch

March 2015

Content Warning: these following few pages speak about suicide. Please only read if you're feeling comfortable and able to do so.

Two weeks later, it was the morning before my final Edinburgh fringe pitch and I was doing some work at CALM. My pitch later that day was with a venue company called Underbelly, where my friend Dan worked in digital marketing, and he had helped beg the producers to at least hear me out regarding a show slot. Underbelly had played host to so many shows I'd loved which combined comedy and theatre, from Guilt N Shame to *Fleabag* to The Rubberbandits. These guys were my last shot at getting a slot for the festival.

The two producers, Marina and Fi, had agreed to give me 45 minutes on a Friday lunchtime in a café next to their office on Mortimer Street in central London, to pitch my little titties off about *Good Grief*.

When I got off the tube, I saw two good luck texts from Daisy and my mum, and then I noticed a few missed calls from Claire. There was an answerphone message from her, and so I stopped at the top of Regent Street.

'Hi Jack. Can you call me, please? We need to talk, so please ring me.'

I immediately thought: It's Olly. I just had this fear that he'd done something and I panic-called my mum. I was about three minutes away from starting the pitch and I just anxiously gargled words at her, along the lines of 'I'm scared my friend Olly has done something bad and I need to do this pitch and it's my last chance.' And, bless my mum, she told me I was being completely stupid and to calm down and focus on what I needed to do.

So that's what I did.

I sat down to start the pitch and Marina and Fi seemed pretty enthused about the show and about me as a performer, but – money was my biggest issue. I thought I had half of what I needed but actually I had a third, and that was already thousands of pounds. Throughout the pitch I was still getting missed calls from Claire and I just knew. I knew it was something bad.

Once it was finished, they said goodbye and I hung around downstairs by their office; I took a deep breath and rang Claire back.

'It's Olly. He's died. Last night. He took his own life and I'm just calling to let you know.' And then she burst into tears and I was just numb. She told me to come up to her guardianship to see her and some of Olly's friends, to just be together.

The pitch

As I hung up the call, I could feel my legs turn heavy, like sandbags. I couldn't walk. I told my friend Dan who worked there what had happened and 15 minutes later Marina the Underbelly producer found me, still awkwardly outside their office. I just didn't know what to do with myself, I was in absolute, total shock, yet at the same time devastated because I felt like I'd seen it coming.

I felt like I'd heard Claire's phone call in my mind before, telling me his demons had won and he'd done it.

Marina hugged me outside the office and we shed a little tear. She said she'll walk me to the station, but I told her I was fine to get there alone.

And then she said, 'Just to let you know, we love the show. In the ten minutes we've been back in the office we've already found you a slot. Four o'clock in the Delhi Belly venue. It's the smallest capacity we have, but we think it would be perfect, and don't worry about the money just yet. We will help you out, you can crowdfund it and we can make it work.'

I feel like this particular moment will stay with me for the rest of my life: getting the worst, most devastating news and the best news I'd been hoping and dreaming of for months, all in the same 15-minute time frame.

I left the office and got the tube up to Claire's.

When I arrived at Claire's guardianship in Camden, Olly's friends Jim and Alisha were already there and we all sat on the rooftop of her building, which was directly opposite the Roundhouse. It was a beautiful sunny day for March, and we sat and just stared out at all of London. Everything felt so calm and so quiet.

We were all in total shock. No one was crying or screaming, we were just paralysed by the fact that he'd actually done it. He'd gone.

We shared our favourite memories of him, what we would miss. His crooked-teeth smile, his penchant for a can of Red Stripe, his flirty wink. I was going to miss all of his little idiosyncrasies that reminded me how sweet he was. How, when I first met him, I cast him aside as a lad's lad, when really he was sensitive and caring and smarter than most men I knew.

I thought about how, in less than one year, my uncle, my nan and Olly had all just gone. All so sudden. For that year, all I had been doing was writing a show about grief sat at the Roundhouse, which I was now looking out at. And everything just felt so surreal and strange and like nothing made any sense. Which, at its core, is the feeling of grief.

To break the tension I told them the good news that I'd finally got my show programmed. They said well done, but it all felt bittersweet.

Twenty or so minutes passed and then I got a phone call from the teaching agency offering me work the next week at a primary school near Morden. I accepted the job.

Shamil

March 2015

Monday morning. I rocked up to this small Catholic primary school wearing a blazer perhaps three chest sizes too tight. I looked like Jane McDonald singing on a cruise, very upright, bit wobbly, tits pushed up and – one could say – *very sexy*.

I was assigned a Year 2 class taught by Miss Bridges, a very abrupt woman in her late thirties from Perth, Australia, who gave off quite a scary Marine Le Pen vibe. Soon enough, the reason why I was at the school became very clear as Miss Bridges sat me next to a Jordanian boy called Shamil. He didn't speak English very well, was relatively misbehaved, and she suspected that he wouldn't listen to women, and she wanted a guy to 'Sort that out, OK?'

Shamil is six. He likes writing, football and looking disapprovingly at my haircut. Another boy called Rupert kept calling me 'Mrs Rooke' and then one of the girls, Ciara, runs up to me and asks, 'Are you a girl or a boy?' When I say I'm a boy, she runs back to her table and says, 'She's a boy!'

Weirdly, Shamil, who supposedly doesn't speak to women, is the only one convinced that I'm not one.

And so I spent the week after Olly's death working at this school and it saved me, to be honest. It gave me focus, a task at hand and the chance to earn a bit of money to put towards Edinburgh.

On my last day, Miss Bridges set a literacy poetry task. The children were to write a poem about Easter. Shamil couldn't care less and stayed reliably silent. He rarely ever spoke in class, only ever using very basic English with me when we were kicking a ball around in the playground.

And so, sat on tiny primary school chairs, I wrote Shamil a poem about how he should talk more, to both boys and girls. And slowly, in his own time, he wrote a poem, but he got really upset and frustrated when he didn't know certain words in English. He didn't always feel able to say how he felt.

And the irony was that I spent the week after Olly's death at a primary school where I was pretty much there to help a little boy who was really very, very sad. And he was trying his hardest to carry on, kicking around a sponge ball and putting up with some judgemental Aussie woman thinking he's useless. On my last day, I gave him a pack of Maoams because I just didn't care if it was naughty. I was also walking around this school playground feeling very sad.

I got home and, after a week of not crying, I just burst into tears. They tumbled out of me, getting louder and louder and more and more reminiscent of Jimmy Carr's laugh. And of course a property guardianship with paper-thin walls is not the best place to grieve. It is not somewhere you can safely let out your emotions with any sense of privacy. As I was crying so loudly, Daisy ran into my room in a sexy outfit mid-way through a camming session, wearing what seemed to be a Japanese kimono, fulfilling some bloke's sexual fantasy for money at the expense of mild cultural appropriation.

And Daisy just held me on my bed and let me cry. She let me shout out all the anger – some of it, if I'm being truly honest, felt almost directed at Olly. I screamed 'You stupid selfish bastard' into my pillow, despite knowing that his death wasn't selfish or stupid at all.

I knew so much about the issue of suicide because of all the work, fundraising and volunteering I'd done for CALM and none of it gave me any solace when I was directly affected by it. I had spoken about the issue with a level of distance that meant it didn't puncture my stomach, whereas now it did. Now it had the ability to floor me, steal my mind away into the caverns of what-ifs. What if I had seen him more those last seven months? What if I had called him every week? What if I'd gone down to Chichester, not left it as a vague plan for 'the spring'? What if I'd been less obsessed with writing a bloody comedy show and had focused more on the fact that when I last saw him he was manic and vulnerable and needed support? And all we had done was send texts.

Daisy told me, sweetly and kindly, as she would many times, that the what-ifs were total bullshit. That there was nothing me, Claire, Jim, Lewis, Tom or anyone could do if someone was that consumed with sadness.

And Daisy just held me as I finished crying. A good half-hour passed of just being sat there, pouring it all out. And then, just as I was finishing, I looked up from our hug and I realised she was wearing sparkly nipple tassles. I burst out laughing.

'Well, they're amazing!'

'I know they are,' she smiled.

We got into bed and ordered a fancy Chinese from the MSG-free place down the road.

goodbye

March–August 2015

Three weeks later, Lewis was driving me, Lily and Tom down to the south coast for Olly's funeral. It was being held at a church in Bognor, near to the seaside Butlins resort I used to go to as a kid.

As we drove closer to the coast, I could feel my chest getting tighter and tighter. I was sweating buckets, sat in the front with the windows down on a wet rainy day in March. And then I realised that I was having an almighty panic attack.

Lewis stopped the car at a petrol station and I just stood, hands on the roof, leaning over the car and trying to breathe.

Lily tried to calm me down, telling me to sip water, like a school nurse at break time. Lewis reminded me that we needed to get moving or else we'd be late. But it all just dawned on me as we'd got closer and closer to the sea.

Back in the car for the last 20 minutes of the drive, I told them we needed to do something to take my mind off it. Tom and Lily started playing this game where you say a celebrity's name and then the next person has to say a name beginning with the first letter of the previous celebrity's surname. If it's an alliterative name, you win a point. This was enough to get me through the journey and into the car park of the church.

Walking into the funeral of a twenty-seven-year-old is horrendous. Seeing young people grieving in ways that I had only ever seen from people double, or three times, that age felt so traumatic. I felt broken that day, but I knew we needed to celebrate him as best as we could.

I remember Olly's ex-girlfriend giving the most incredible speech during his service, with such strength and humour, about what a caring, kind boy Olly was.

And then my next memory is of leaving the chapel and suddenly not feeling so strong any more.

I couldn't watch the burial.

I couldn't face it, so Lily and I just sat alone on a bench. We walked down Bognor seafront, got fish and chips and then drove back home.

And for those months after, I pushed Olly to the back of my mind. I just couldn't go there yet. I asked everyone to never tell me any details about his passing. I didn't want to know how he did it, because, after my dissertation, I knew that I wouldn't want the image in my mind.

I didn't want to know what was in his suicide letter.

I didn't want to know any reasons that he had given.

I just wanted to focus on earning the money to make the best possible show for Edinburgh.

I just wanted, for a brief moment, to forget.

how to help someone bereaved by a suicide

The suicide of a loved one can often feel like a series of failures. It leaves failure dripping from the lips of those who loved someone who's gone. It leaves the aftertaste of failure in the mouths of friends, relatives, partners, ex-partners, colleagues and peers. The what-if questions run races around your head at night. 'What if I'd just ...' 'How did I fail to notice ...' 'Why didn't I say ... '

Suicide highlights the failures in our society, our media, our government, our health services and all the ways in which we effectively try to protect the people who are the most vulnerable.

And in the hardest moments, suicide feels like a failure of the love we have for those we care about. But what I've learnt since Olly's passing is that this failure isn't true.

Many of the very intense and complex feelings attached to the tragedy of suicide are also entangled in the stigma and shame present in some cultures. It's so important to defeat this stigma and to understand that, within all these failures, no one is ever solely to blame. There is never one specific reason why someone has felt so low they have taken their own life. It's often a long-term battle and, if you have tried countless times to support someone after they've made numerous attempts, yet they still choose to eventually take their own life, the difficult feelings left behind can be devastating and almost impossible to accept.

Therefore, it is so important that, if you're trying to support someone bereaved by a suicide, you understand some of these difficult feelings and the nuances of them.

1 Numbness and denial.

This was my first emotion. A feeling of complete nothingness. Losing Olly was very different to when I'd lost my dad and my nan because then I had immediately felt the pain and heartbreak of saying goodbye. But when I heard about Olly I felt so empty, exhausted almost. I felt like I had been robbed of the opportunity to say goodbye, the chance to hang out after nine months of not seeing each other. I felt that I just wasn't done with him yet. To the people around me I looked like I was coping quite well. But behind that numbness, thinking about Olly was consuming all my inner thoughts, but I just couldn't articulate that for a quite a while.

I think it is so important to allow someone to experience this numbness and just let them know you're there for when they finally feel ready and can let some of those contained emotions out.

In this numbness there was, for me, an element of denial. Not necessarily denial that Olly had taken his own life, but I wanted with all my heart to believe it was just a mistake. That he probably did not intend to do it. I clung on to this for a while after he died and it did not do me any good. I would encourage anyone bereaved by suicide to try not to question what anyone's motivations were, or how certain their intent. Fixating on this totally exhausted me, and ultimately none of us will ever truly discover the full answer, which is part of why suicide feels like such a hard thing to deal with.

2 Questioning and shame.

Part of my denial was formed by a heavy dose of rhetorical questions that swirled around my head thick and fast, leaving me in a daze or interrupting any seemingly normal thought track to wonder why he was gone. The smallest thing, reminder or everyday phrase could trigger this in me. I asked myself over and over, 'I wonder what the real reason was? I wonder what had actually happened? What if we had all just ... ?' etc.

This level of questioning particularly doesn't help in that initial period of bereavement. So often in my work for CALM I would speak to people who'd also lost young male friends or relatives and quite often I'd hear people say, 'No one knew he was struggling.' But me and Olly had spoken on a few occasions about our mental wellbeing, I knew that he'd experienced suicidal ideation before and yet this didn't make it any easier to accept his eventual death. It made it in many ways ten times harder because I just questioned everything I'd ever done or said, with harsh self-criticism.

'How can I be an ambassador of a male suicide prevention charity, yet I've just lost a male friend to suicide?'

I felt ashamed, that I'd failed him almost, even though I knew that I was there for him whenever he needed a chat at uni. Asking questions often won't bring answers that will help or bring peace to the bereaved. Instead they can become fixations or cause feelings of guilt that prevent the healing process. As someone trying to support a loved one bereaved by suicide, it's important to try to listen to these questions and get the person to understand which ones are worth asking and which ones they need to find a way to stop going over and over in their heads. Those 'what if' questions will only ever result in someone torturing themselves, so try to get them away from any hypotheticals.

3 Anger.

There was a real anger that was generally dormant in my emotions and then, in certain moments, I'd descend into a pure rage against the world, against myself and, if I'm being totally honest, even against Olly. As I mentioned earlier – with screaming into my pillow, 'You selfish prick!' – I sometimes misdirected anger at him in moments of distress.

I categorically, 100 per cent knew in my heart that Olly's suicide was *not* a selfish act. I'd written parts of my dissertation about the dangerous stigmas attached to suicide, and my volunteering work with CALM involved trying to educate people about how suicide isn't selfish. But when feeling vulnerable, when the pain and sadness of such a loss affects your judgement, these are the moments where you may feel anger. Regretfully, I sometimes felt angry at Olly for doing it. For causing his friends even closer to him, like Claire, to go through so much loss and pain. She didn't deserve this, but neither did Olly deserve to struggle with such severe mental illness.

I learnt that this was anger I needed to work through with patience, trying to release those difficult emotions by doing something positive with them, for example putting on fundraisers for CALM or writing down any confused feelings, channelling them into a creative outlet. Never underestimate the benefits of a blank sheet of paper to just get everything out on. Also, anger is something very important to get people to speak about in any therapy or counselling, because it can be the source of much self-sabotaging and damaging behaviour.

4 **Rejection and loneliness.**

I didn't feel this so much, but I have spoken to many people who, after the suicide of a loved one, feel a palpable sense of isolation and rejection. They can question why they weren't enough for someone to stay. This, to me, definitely feels like a rational train of thought, but I also think it's crucial to recognise, despite the grief, that the person you've lost is not just the mental illness or demons that led to the reason they're gone. No one in their right mind who is in a good or stable place in their life wants to abandon their loved ones; it is their own pain and suffering they want to escape from.

I believe quite passionately that it's important to sensitively remind someone who is bereaved of the loving bond they had with the person who's gone. Despite the traumatic and tragic way in which they left, I still believe we have to openly celebrate and cherish those people and the moments of happiness we shared with them. I try to do this with my friends all the time, cheersing a round down the pub to Olly or making sure to share funny stories of him whenever the feeling comes up. I don't want to forget the huge impact he had on me in the short few years I knew him.

5 Relief and guilt.

I have also heard from many bereaved people who feel guilty over a sense of relief that they experience when a person has finally 'done it'. If someone had been deeply troubled for a long time, it makes sense that, though we would never want someone to take their own life, there may still be a valid feeling of relief that they're at peace. I definitely felt this when I've lost relatives to physical illness – that release of tight knots of energy in your stomach when you know someone you love is no longer in pain. I don't think anyone should beat themselves up or see themselves as selfish for feeling that when it comes to suicide. A big part of being bereaved by a suicide is trying to overcome personal guilt and accept what has happened. Even if the bereaved person can never accept the reasons why or the circumstances of how they lost someone, it is important to help them to accept that the person they loved has gone.

6 Judgement and stigma.

Sadly, despite mental health conversations reaching an all-time high in the UK, old-fashioned stigmas and judgements persist, perhaps connected to certain cultures, religious beliefs or prejudices, that mean people are still dismissive of those who have taken their own life or experience severe mental illness. I think you must try as best you can to get bereaved people to ignore this stigma and, at the same time, help to fight it by spreading your own awareness and compassion within your community. We can't rewrite scriptures or history, but we can change the words we use and we can be kinder. Again, I'd really recommend reading the Samaritans' media guidelines on suicide reporting as I think they give really important information on how we should all sensitively and appropriately talk about suicide in our society.

I've said this sooo many times in this book, but I really believe that the best way to support someone going through this wide range of complex emotions is to just make sure you're there and available to listen. Once you've allowed someone the proper space to let out their feelings, don't be afraid to then engage in difficult conversations or to openly say the name of the person who has died. Be sure to let them know that there is professional support available for those bereaved by suicide, which can be accessed by contacting a charity like Papyrus or CALM, visiting your GP for NHS mental health services or, if you're financially able to, by sourcing a private specialist bereavement counsellor.

On a personal level, I really believe that planning or doing something for charity, which feels conducive to something positive being achieved or to preventing any more people going through the same pain, can massively help someone affected by suicide. It might feel daunting, but there are things you can do that can help.

Lastly, I feel it's important to add that a suicide can be just as draining and still very affecting even if you yourself aren't directly connected to the person who's died. Even just being the loved one of someone bereaved by a suicide can feel exhausting and traumatic. It is one of the worst tragedies of the human experience and it's important to check in with yourself on how talking about it is affecting you. It certainly has taken its toll on me over the years, even before Olly died, when I was just volunteering at CALM. It's a tricky topic to discuss and then try to feel normal or positive or even just OK afterwards.

Again, as I've said before, when trying to support a bereaved person, it can be very easy to feel like you're doing things wrong or that you aren't doing enough, but I really believe there is no definitively correct way. Whilst I've tried to make sure the tips and ideas I've given in this book on how best to support someone in midst of an emotionally challenging time cover most situations, when it comes to the aftermath of a suicide, it does really completely depend on the person affected. Remember that it is not your fault if they aren't coping. This is something I have had to realise as someone who has been directly affected by a suicide and has also watched a friend go through that loss. You can't magic away someone else's pain, you just have to be there, ready to listen, and at the same time make sure that you are looking after yourself too, so you don't feel overwhelmed or under too much pressure.

You are going to be needed in the darkest moments of someone's grief, but I promise the happier times do start to come back. No matter how hard it can feel for someone to accept a suicide, life goes on, and people adapt and grow.

Ultimately, it's important that we collectively make sure we don't see suicide as this massive failure but as something that we can tackle, accept, educate people about, and prevent from feeling like a valid option to the people we love in times of crisis.

good grief, Edinburgh 2015

August 2015

After the funeral and initial few months of grief, going up to the Edinburgh Fringe Festival and having something positive to focus my energies on had helped me massively. Even though the show was essentially me speaking for an hour in front of total strangers about two other bereavements, it was cathartic. I felt very lucky being able to see and hear my nan on film every single time I performed the show. It kind of felt like she was still with me, saving me from spiralling into a depressive episode about Olly that I knew was waiting, somewhere in my head, ready to escalate when I gave it the breathing space to do so.

I couldn't face hosting Bang Said the Gun after Olly passed, so I stepped back from the night to focus solely on preparing for the fringe. My friend Gabriel from *Guilt and Shame* agreed to direct the show and together we tried to shape *Good Grief* into the best possible debut hour for the Edinburgh audience. But it was all a huge risk. I was really in quite a vulnerable place, spending so much money and investing so much of my energy into something that could quite easily flop, with no publicity campaign or expensive marketing behind me.

We arrived at the festival and Blu-Tacked about seventy posters all around Edinburgh's cafés, kebab shops, arts venues, pubs and the odd telephone box and then we got the show up on its feet, testing that all the projections worked in the venue. There was a tiny dressing room for around forty performers to share, which was essentially just a dripping damp cave in a multi-story car park with black curtains hung up to provide some sense of 'privacy' and 'glamour'.

My job before every show was to ensure the right amount of Soreen slices had been cut and buttered to give out to the audience members. On the day we opened, I had prepped forty slices of buttered Soreen and we had a grand audience of twelve people. Rest assured I offered double portions.

I guess the low audience figures were mainly because no one knew who I was and my show was slam bang in the middle of the afternoon and all about death – it wasn't necessarily the easiest sell. However, about six shows in, my first review came out. A theatre blog I'd never even heard of gave me a glowing five stars and I was absolutely jumping for joy. The next day another reviewer came in, this time from a better-known performing arts review site called Broadway Baby – it was five stars again. I started plastering paper strips with five-star emojis all over my very shoddy Edinburgh posters, and noticed that my sales began to reach the thirty-five/forty ticket mark, which I was over the moon with.

Audiences started to comment after shows on how much they loved getting to know my nan and how heartbreaking yet sweet they found her death at the end of the show. Some audience members began to share with me that they had also experienced huge bereavements and had often felt too awkward to open up and talk about it. After shows, whole groups and families of people soon began to wait outside the venue to talk to me, to remember a loved one of theirs or recount an awkwardly funny moment at their aunty's funeral. Some audience members would burst into tears after the show and cry on me for 15 minutes about everything from dead dads to dead dogs and I'd just be there, hugging sobbing strangers on cobbled Edinburgh back streets like some sort of Harry Styles of grief. It was quite mad.

My third review came out at the start of the second week of the festival. It was another five stars, this time from *Gay Times* magazine, an actual national publication. I was eleven shows in out of twenty-five and I had exclusively five-star reviews on my posters. The PR team at my venue then started taking notice of me, and this little solo show in the smallest capacity room of the venue, about a boy and his nan coping with grief, suddenly began to sell out.

Good Grief became one of those rare Edinburgh sleeper hits. The *Guardian* theatre critic Lyn Gardner came in and featured me in the newspaper's 'shows to watch at the fringe' article. There were more crying audience members, and now about three quarters of the crowd would be waiting outside at the end to chat to me. Soon enough, awards judges were coming in to see the show and, by the end of the second week, I had been nominated for the Total Theatre award for best show by an emerging artist. In my mind I was barely even that, I was just some guy who'd just graduated from a media degree and had hosted a rowdy poetry night above a pub. Now I was being celebrated by the actual fringe theatre world of the Edinburgh festival as an 'artist'; it was incredibly exciting and very, very bizarre.

In the final week of *Good Grief*'s run, I received an email from the venue's press office that the *New York Times*' theatre critic wanted to come in and see the show. I was floored. The following day I was added to a 'highlights of the fringe' piece in an international newspaper! The radio commissioner for BBC Comedy came because I'd flyered her and was incredibly positive about the show, and soon enough a meeting was put in for me to pitch *Good Grief* as an adaption for Radio 4.

It just was the best festival experience I could ever have dreamt of. In many ways that month is one of the happiest of my life, even though Olly's loss was never too far from my thoughts. But I really felt like I'd done him proud. I felt like I'd done my nan proud and I'd done my dad proud too. After all the pain of losing them, I'd made something positive out of that grief. I'd made something to commemorate them and to help others by making people laugh and open up about the bullshit awkwardness of it all. And in many ways I felt like I had done fifteen-year-old me proud. I felt like I had finally become more of myself again.

Bridget Jones and the local newspaper

September–December 2015

I returned to London from the month in Edinburgh and I pushed my inconveniently large coffin back up fifty stairs into our weird property guardianship. That same day, we all found out we'd been evicted with two weeks' notice. Over the summer, while I was away, there had been lots of roof parties and boozy blow-outs, and rumours were circulating that two people even had a spot of al-fresco, roof-top intercourse, which was viewed and heard by many of our Hampstead Heath neighbours. George Michael would have been proud as punch, but, sadly, Julie at the property guardianship company gave everyone a bollocking and a measly fortnight to find somewhere new to live.

I'd met a lovely TV producer called Dave in Edinburgh via our mutual friend Vicky. Dave was a dry-witted, curly-haired, chubby gay man – essentially a double of me but a about a decade older and infinitely wiser. We looked like sisters and hit it off immediately. I told him I'd been kicked out my guardianship and he said I could stay in his spare room for two to three weeks whilst I found somewhere to live.

I exclaimed, 'Yes, please, I'd love to come stay!', jumping at the chance to live in an actual habitable environment and not just a room in an office block above a Kwik Fit.

'Where is your flat?' I added.

Dave replied, 'London Bridge, next to Borough Market.'

My jaw dropped. My two to three weeks' stay turned into a four-and-a-half month extended visit. I was living out my long-lasting secret gay dream of being Bridget Jones, a fresh-faced singleton strutting around the artisan cheese-scented lanes of Borough Market whilst living in a top-floor apartment near the train line. I graduated from Blossom Hill white Zinfandel to bottles of dark red Beaujolais, like a twenty-two-year-old middle-aged lady in waiting.

Dave's place immediately felt homely, mainly because it absolutely stank of the cigarettes that my mum chainsmoked every day when I was a kid. 'Cutters Choice rollies or Marlboro Lights, if they haven't got any in the petrol garage'. The flat was at the very top of a building with no lift, which provided me with more than enough daily exercise to bolster my endorphin levels. Dave's spare room also gave me somewhere private to recover from what had been a mad year.

Everything in my life seemed to be going very well. I was going to be putting on the show at an off-West End theatre, some agents were interested in signing me and I had a concrete offer from Radio 4 to adapt *Good Grief* into a 30-minute comedy special.

Around six weeks after I'd moved in to Dave's, in early October, I met up in a pub with Daisy, the infamous webcam girl of my property guardianship. Somehow, three glasses of wine in, we got on to the topic of Olly. She asked me if I ever found out 'how he did it?'

Having written my dissertation on the dangerous reportage of suicide methods, and following my experiences volunteering at CALM, I had told all of my and Olly's mutual friends not to tell me how he had taken his life. I guess that was predominantly because it did not feel relevant to me. The method he had chosen was not something I needed or wanted to know, and I suppose I also just didn't want the image of it in my head.

At Olly's wake I had covered my ears when a few people discussed it. At Halloween, a drunken Claire, dressed in a very low cut 'sexy-scary' catwoman costume, had started to tell me over a two-for-one Sex on the Beach in a cocktail bar that she didn't think Olly meant to kill himself because … But before she could finish her sentence, I stole her catwoman ears, accidentally yanking up her costume and popping open her chest buttons in the process, revealing one of her breasts to the whole table. This did mean, however, that she was completely thrown and it prevented her from telling me any more information.

And then, one night while I was still staying at Dave's but he was away, I googled Olly's name to find some of our old student radio station programmes, just so I could hear his voice. Within the search results was the headline of a news article from a couple months previously, that came from the local newspaper of the town Olly passed away in. It read: *'Graduate from Chichester planning for future before suicide.'*

I clicked on it. The article began describing Olly as 'an aspiring journalist and teacher who hoped to travel to Japan [who] took his own life despite receiving psychiatric help.' It went on to say how he was keen to make progress with his mental health and was very motivated, having been interviewed for teaching positions out in Japan. However, there was some concern he might not be able to take his medication out there, so he'd tried to come off it slowly by reducing his dosage himself and that may have affected his state of mind and mental health in the days before his passing.

It was heartbreaking to read about someone I loved, who I'd met studying journalism, being discussed like another statistic in a news article.

And then, in the very middle of this seemingly standard online piece, it said: *'In March 2015, Oliver died by* [stated the method]. *Recording a conclusion of suicide, a coroner said: "We know he left a suicide letter and it's clear the act he undertook was an intentional act."'*

I was shaking for hours after I read it. I had a panic attack. I felt the four walls of Dave's spare room slowly cave in on me. All the questioning of the method and the reasoning I'd tried to stop my mind from wandering into suddenly felt like it'd cemented itself into my head. I had written a whole dissertation on why this wasn't sensitive media practice and then I ended up experiencing it in my own life. It felt insane but also not at all surprising. A lot of our media don't know how to handle suicide well enough.

The effects this had on me in the weeks after I read it were very strange. I almost began the grieving process again. I would picture him in my sleep undertaking the act and wake up, distressed, crying and feeling so lost. Whilst everything in my professional life was taking off, finding out how just absolutely broke me, because everything I had hoped maybe wasn't the case turned out to be true.

I still try to live my life in the belief that Olly really did want to live. That Olly was trying hard to get better and get on with life. But that this concern over his medication with moving abroad, which resulted in him trying to gradually lower his dosage, all played a part in the reasons why he is no longer here.

I had so badly hoped it was a mistake – an attempt he didn't want to succeed – but discovering there was a letter and a coroner's conclusion that it was intentional just made me want to continue trying to support CALM as best as I could. I knew I needed to focus on making work and creating projects to help spread awareness of suicide prevention, and I guess, in some ways, to make myself feel like I was doing something positive in his memory.

success and failure

2016 and 2017

Over the following two years, lots of cool, wonderful and brilliant things happened in my life. I signed with an agent and got a commission to write a follow-up Edinburgh show for Fringe 2017 called *Happy Hour,* about young male suicide. I felt very lucky to be given opportunities to make work about issues I cared about. I went from being the phone operator at Radio 1's *Surgery* programme to being their on-air expert in bereavement and mental health, which led to getting a green light to present my very first TV documentary, a three-part series for BBC Three called *Happy Man*, about alternative, free mental wellbeing practices that can help young people in a mental health crisis. My dream had always been to be the fat gay Stacey Dooley and, at last, it was happening!

On the outside, everything was going well, yet underneath it all, I was really quite miserable. I was back living at my mum's and just powering through, almost sinisterly switching between 'tits 'n' teeth Jack' to an emotionally crumbling crying mess behind closed doors.

I found making the documentary difficult at times. What I thought it was going to be when I initially developed the idea wasn't quite what we ended up making, which can happen very easily in the process of making TV, as programmes shape and refine themselves. In my mind, the episodes could have touched more on mental health cuts and the state of services available for young people. There was one scene that didn't make the final edits, which showed me laying flowers and a can of Red Stripe at Olly's graveside and saying how I felt he would still be here had there been more services in Early Intervention to help him at a younger age. A big part of making TV is compromise and I knew that I just had to trust that the show would help lots of young viewers regardless of what did or didn't make the final cut. And there were still some brilliant experiences in making the project which I'm incredibly grateful for.

I went to interview a drag queen who had just come out of prison and was changing their life around, then I went for a dip with a nineteen-year-old guy in Scotland who was using cold-water swimming in freezing cold lakes to tackle his depression and then, in the final episode, I got (semi) naked for a life drawing class to look at the issue of body image.

However, despite how lucky I felt, I also look back on these two years of my life and realise that, deep down, I was very depressed and keeping it incredibly concealed, until I couldn't any longer. It had been such an intense few years since leaving the safe confines of my university flat in West Hampstead, where my main worry had been whether or not I'd get to the reduced food aisle in Tesco in time to nab the best stuff.

My mum began to get incredibly worried about me when I was filming the show, as I started becoming increasingly more emotionally erratic. I would cry all morning, literally bawling about how I didn't know why I felt so sad, but I just felt completely overwhelmed by everything, and then I'd get a text that a car was waiting outside to take me to a day of filming. It was dangerous and I knew that the workload was really starting to get to me, but each time I'd remind myself that it was exposure and money. I'd been so skint after university and there was no parent able to financially support me as I got on my feet in adult life, and somehow I'd now found this career. I had to take any financial stability where I could get it, but it was essentially me being sad for pay. There were moments during this time when I felt like a bit of a fraud, becoming some poster child for young male mental health when really I was struggling myself.

When I finally practised what I preached and told BBC Three about how I was feeling, they organised a therapist for me for a few sessions. Before our first session the therapist started following me on Twitter and googled me and this just felt like it undermined the reasons why I needed a therapist. I wanted someone to respect some sense of my right to anonymity in the therapy room and who didn't have a preconceived idea of what I'd been through based on what was on the internet. At the time it felt embarrassing, and like it stripped me of the chance to divulge my own story and explain what had happened in my latter teen years. I also think it made me feel really anxious, because the public-facing personality that I was on Twitter, tweeting jokes about fancying my friends' hot dads, was not the person I wanted to present in the privacy of a therapy room to someone I desperately wanted to help me with my private turmoil. In the end, I didn't go to more than two sessions because I just didn't feel like the style of talking therapy was going to work for me. I'd say now that I gave up far too soon, but I just didn't think I needed CBT; I thought I needed more analytical psychotherapy into my relationships, past traumas and how they were contributing to my mental health problems.

I began to fall even more into a cycle of depression. I began drinking more, lots more, and not nice bottles of red wine at Dave's flat but the sort of booze you drink when you're feeling miserable as fuck. I had generally been a 'go big or go Appletiser' kind of drinker – I wouldn't just have an alcoholic drink at the end of a day and generally only drank if I was going on a night out or was at a party. Gradually I began buying mini-bottles of red wine at 2.30pm in Tesco Metro with my meal deal alongside.

Along with my increase in drinking, I started going to gay clubs completely on my own. I'd go on to Grindr in clubs and, instead of going around chatting to people, I would just tap the app and up came an Argos catalogue of gays, in stock, ready for collection. I'd put myself in vulnerable situations, emotionally, and had some rather beige transactional hook-ups, the sort that leave you feeling a bit empty inside. Then

I'd find myself wandering aimlessly around central London late at night. There were so many times I would walk from a club called XXL on the South Bank and I'd stumble drunk across Blackfriars Bridge, thinking about what would happen if I just ended it all. Then the next day I would just go to work and put on a big grin.

One evening, in the winter of 2016, I was booked to be on the closing panel talk for the Being a Man Festival at the Southbank Centre. The talk was to around 200 people, who'd been to numerous events at the festival, about what society could do to better understand the challenges facing men today. During one anecdote I was telling, I made a casual remark mentioning how I'd once dated a guy who always listened to rain sounds every night, which I found highly off-putting so I'd try to turn it off once he was asleep, but he'd immediately wake up. People laughed, but it was just a tiny throwaway remark in a much wider discussion.

Then, at the end of the talk, Jude Kelly, former artistic director of the Southbank Centre, who was chairing the panel, asked for questions from the audience. I'd expected this to be one of those standard Q&As where an audience member gets hold of a roaming microphone and shares a story about themselves without actually asking a single question. We've all been there.

Except the first person to ask was a man, perhaps in his early forties, who stood up and looked dead straight at me, saying into the roaming mic: 'I want to know why the Southbank Centre has decided to book so many gay panellists across this festival when only 2 per cent of the world is gay, therefore it's not a perspective 98 per cent of men care to hear.'

Audience members gasped, the room went deadly silent. Jude sat forward and asked him to clarify his point, remarking that his statistics didn't make sense.

The lovely gentleman with the microphone then kindly elaborated, saying that he felt that, by the Southbank Centre hosting so many gay speakers (there were only two on this panel), it was 'normalising and promoting homosexuality' and the festival would have been, in his words, 'more masculine' had they not got so many of us lot on stage.

This was the first time as an adult that I'd felt directly and publicly embarrassed by a someone being homophobic. I was trapped, sat in the middle of a stage behind a microphone, with 200 pairs of eyes looking at me, waiting for a response. It took me straight back to Year 10 when Luke Stainers mouthed the word 'faggot' at me in Mr Adewolo's maths class. However, this man, stood up in a relatively placid middle-class arts venue, did not look like the nasty homophobe I'd imagined held these opinions. He looked kind, sweet, well dressed and actually remarkably like the footballer John Barnes – which was a real shame because I love John Barnes!

And so I stood up and in retaliation I started belting out Elton's John's 'Electricity' from the *Billy Elliot* musical as loudly as I could … nah, I'm joking. I completely froze and just tried to stop my knees from trembling. I had no idea what to say.

At twenty-three years old, not only had I never had an adult be homophobic towards me, but I hadn't expected to experience it for the first time whilst on stage at an arts festival, as opposed to, say, Watford High Street McDonald's at 3am when I was pretending to deep throat a Chicken Select for someone's Instagram story.

Thankfully, Jude was very clever and told the lovely homophobe that she would take all of the audience's questions straight away and then we'd answer them one by one. This bought me time so I could think up my reply, almost as if Jude was telepathically communicating to me, 'You've got this, lad! I believe in you!'

As the other speakers on the panel answered other audience questions, some of them briefly addressed the first guy's bizarre accusations and defended the Southbank Centre for booking real life gay men who could speak words (I later found out there were only a handful of gays actually booked to speak across the whole festival). However, I could see that everyone in the room of 200 people was sat waiting for my reply. Jude rather cleverly left his question till last and, soon enough, it was my turn.

I sat up straight and said, 'Hello. I'm Jack. I've been booked today on this Being a Man panel because I'm making a BBC Three series about male mental health called *Happy Man* about losing my male parent at fifteen and losing a close male friend to suicide last year and being a volunteer for a male suicide prevention charity called CALM. The producers booking me for this event didn't even know I'm gay because I'm not really "out out", as of yet. Even my mum doesn't really know the way I identify, mainly because my sexuality has not influenced my identity in the more prominent ways that bereavement and class have done. And, even if it had, me being gay wouldn't be a problem to anyone who was secure in themselves. So I think, if anything, considering what I've been through, I'm probably the most qualified male to be on this panel, even with the whole big fat gay thing going on!'

As the audience whooped, clapped and cheered my response, I then stood up and sang Elton John's 'Electricity' as loudly as I ... Nah, I'm still joking. I just got a lovely supportive round of applause and the panel discussion ended. The homophobic man just nodded and, as the talk packed down, I watched him as he got up, put his navy blue coat on, wrapped a nice grey scarf around his neck, picked up his tote bag and went to leave the room. And I was so angry that he could just do that. That he could say something so loaded and shitty and then just walk out the door. But, thankfully, before he could exit, a mini-army of women started giving him a mouthful, one of them saying, 'Well your question was absolute fucking bullshit, mate. Why?'

I smiled and left via another door. As soon I was outside I felt myself gasping for air. Some of my fellow panellists and staff at the Southbank checked that I was OK and then I got the train home to my mum's house. That night I couldn't sleep, but I felt really proud of myself because, in so many moments of my life, I hadn't felt like I was confident or smart enough to articulate my sexuality and at last I'd done that. All it took was some good old-fashioned homophobic denial of my right to speak on a bloody arts panel. It's almost too cringey and clichéd to write about, but I thought it relevant.

I posted about the homophobic man on Facebook around 3am that night, which meant publicly coming out to whoever on my friends list I hadn't told, but it wasn't like a big 'coming out', it was more of a general announcement, like when a flight's been cancelled. Nothing big, just a reminder that homophobes are massive losers. The post got 912 likes, which was enough to give me a nice serotonin boost for the day.

Then the next day I told my mum and she just hugged me, told me to ignore any homophobic bastards and that she would always be happy with whoever I ended up with, so long as I was happy.

'I'll always love you, just as long as you never delete the series record for *Poldark* or *Call the Midwife*!' she joked, as we held hands. I felt this huge weight roll off my shoulders, after all those years of worrying or lying about myself. All those years as a kid where I was anxious I wasn't enough of a boy or a lad, all seemed to slowly dissipate. From this moment onwards I just stopped giving a shit.

Mum added, 'Even if you murdered someone, I'd probably still love you. It'd be bloody hard and I probably wouldn't like you very much, but I'd still always love ya!'

I replied to her, still holding hands, 'Same, but let's not murder anyone, because I have a TV show coming out soon.'

And we agreed to never hypothetically kill ever again.

mental breakdown cover

2017/2018

When the BBC Three series finally came out in April 2017, I began to feel quite overwhelmed. The trailer for the show garnered over 5 million views on Facebook, with hundreds of thousands of shares and retweets. My inboxes on all my social media were bombarded by messages from young people who were struggling, who either wanted to share their story or even to admit to me they were suicidal. I received harrowing messages from kids who kept ropes under their beds, who had planned numerous methods of suicide in case they one day felt they could no longer cope.

No one really prepared me for this onslaught of messages and it often left me in fits of sheer terror and panic. I knew how to hug a crying audience member after a performance of *Good Grief* and I knew how to speak to young people on Radio 1 calling in with stress or anxiety issues and I knew how to reach out to my loved ones who I was worried about – but I did not know how to cope with vulnerable people telling me from behind a screen that they'd watched my show and they wanted to kill themselves.

The irony of this being that, in episode 1 of *Happy Man*, I drove round London, with a megaphone, hanging out the window of a vehicle recovery truck which had huge LED screens on the side displaying the words 'Do You Have Mental Breakdown Cover?' Then I'd shout this question at total strangers on the streets of Covent Garden from the passenger window, whilst never actually asking myself this question.

In the summer of 2017, I started to experience the beginnings of a breakdown at the Edinburgh Fringe festival, where I was doing my second show, *Happy Hour*, about male suicide. I'd had that dream Edinburgh festival experience in 2015, and this time round the show still did well, with lots of five- and four-star reviews and an award nomination from the Mental Health Foundation, but I personally didn't cope well performing hard stories about losing Olly every day. It was too much. I would cry for hours on the phone to friends back in London or irrationally beg the producers to let me go home for a couple of days to see my mum. It was the longest time of my whole life that I had spent away from her and that was enough for my anxieties to begin spiralling out of control.

I remember doing one show where I had cried the whole afternoon before the performance and then went on stage with no energy and forgot my lines about a quarter of the way through. Afterwards, I completely fell to pieces backstage. A reviewer saw it and gave the show a two-star review. I was devastated and realised that I just couldn't carry on doing it.

I cancelled performing *Happy Hour* in London when I returned home and I fell further into spirals of anxiety and paranoia. I told myself that I'd somehow ruined my career, the paranoid anxiety starting to fully take hold of my mind as I was drinking more, having more pointless hook-ups and completely driving myself into a rut of full-on self-sabotage.

It all came to a head around the end of 2017, when I got caught, drunk, shoplifting a secret santa present in a cheap clothes shop. Completely numb and out of it, I was taken upstairs to a detention room, with an excited security guard commenting, 'Well, you don't look like a tea leaf!'

I was just completely lost and it was a huge cry for help. The total value of the items I'd stolen was around £7, not enough for a police inquiry but enough to get me slapped with a £100 fine.

Getting caught drunk, doing something illegal and immensely embarrassing, triggered that felt long overdue by the start of 2018. For nearly a whole month crippling anxiety had me bed bound, making only the odd visit to the bathroom for a poo or going downstairs to get a glass of water. I lost over a stone in weight.

I had spoken to so many people with anxiety disorder in the previous seven years and yet I'd just nodded with sympathy at how bad it was. I guess I thought anxiety was just a really bad case of the nerves, but once afflicted with it on a severe level I realised it was absolute hell. It was like being trapped on a ship, the HMS *Anxious Breakdown*, and I just had to ride each wave until there was a period of stillness again.

Throughout the whole two years of making a documentary and writing a show about suicide, I had only had two actual therapy sessions with someone who I didn't feel was at all right to help me. But now I tried everything to make myself feel better. I went to an incredibly expensive hypnotherapy session at a boutique Neal's Yard therapy centre, where I mainly spent 35 minutes sniffing seventy different varieties of herbal oils and essences to help me 'go under', and then I was far too anxious to actually complete the therapy properly. That was a waste of £200.

Then I had some therapy over the phone, which slightly helped, even if it was just the placebo effect of feeling that by speaking to a therapist I was curing myself, but in reality I gave up on those sessions far too soon as well. My GP gave me the option of starting medication, but I decided against it. I think probably due to fears attached to Olly's death and the article about him trying to come off his meds without proper supervision.

In the end, what helped me was talking to my loved ones and just starting to look after myself. I used to joke that self-care to me was just having a poo when you first felt it coming. But once I really was in a difficult period, I started to realise that self-care wasn't just a gimmick but something very important in allowing people to function in their daily life. I started doing some exercise each week. I would spend time sitting alone in a quiet room and reflecting, which was like my own version of meditating, but it involved having an Options low-fat hot chocolate.

Gradually, with some time out, a period of sobriety and the deletion of anything that even resembled a gay dating or hook-up app, I started to feel much happier. Not completely out of the woods, but like I was on the right road out of the dark period in my head.

By the end of summer 2018, I signed this book deal, as well as a script commission to write and film a sitcom pilot called *Big Boys* – based on a gay guy and a straight guy becoming best mates at uni. I'd stopped putting myself on TV talking about depressing topics or being a poster child for sad men. Instead I spent this time falling back into just writing again, which has always been my favourite form of catharsis. It's how I became such good friends with Olly in the first place and it's how I've coped after anything awful that's ever happened to me.

Now, as I finish writing this book, I'm in a much better place, albeit with different sorts of challenges. At twenty-five, I feel like I understand my own mental health much better and what I need from my friends, family and work life.

So much of understanding one's mental health is just about figuring out what works specifically for you, what can make you feel worse, what you want to avoid and the long-term solutions that can make you feel you can access the right support.

For me, it's always been about having that creative outlet, because I still write lines of words and feelings into notebooks or my iPhone notes about my dad. I still think about my nan and the gifts she's given me. And I still think about all the wise and kind advice Olly said to me.

Writing this book has been incredibly hard in many ways yet completely cathartic, all in one. It's been emotionally tough thinking back to the times when I felt too scared to ask Olly about his mental state in case I wasn't good enough or couldn't help him properly. Ultimately, though, what I have realised in the five years he's been gone is that I was always good enough. Not because I worked for CALM or because I had experienced my own mental health issues, but just because I loved him.

My last advice guide is, in many ways, a manifesto for the future. It's kind of a 'How to help save people at their most vulnerable' and a 'How to be a mental health activist that demands both more talking and more action'!

After changing the title numerous times of this final guide, I have settled on what feels like the most important message of all: 'How not to be scared'.

how not to be scared

I began this book describing how fear and love operate on the same level. It's the reason why many heterosexual parents love their kids dearly but can feel incredibly scared for them if they come out as LGBTQ+, in case they get bullied or experience prejudice and cruelty. Fear is the reason why sometimes we tell our loved ones to 'cheer the fuck up' when really we just want them to be safe and get better . We can all feel driven by fear.

But I think we have to be stronger and fight more of these fears, because they can result in silence and a lack of action in helping people who really need it. And, actually, there are a lot of brave people and initiatives out there, all listed below, which need us to support and join them in tackling this fear and, ultimately, saving more people's lives.

1 Don't be scared to get it wrong.

We all fuck up! We all have moments where we make the worst mistakes. Never be frightened that you'll say the wrong thing because, in the end, saying something is better than saying nothing at all. You can even admit to someone that you don't know what the best thing to say is, but that you're there to listen.

If speaking is something you find difficult, then write someone you care about a letter or an email or a long text explaining how you want to be there for them. Supporting someone doesn't have to be scary; just remember to be compassionate and non-judgemental and put yourself in other people's shoes.

2 Mental health first aid.

A few years back, I came across the term 'mental health first aid'. It's the same as physical first aid, but rather than learning about heart compressions and how to make a sling from a scarf, you can get training to equip you to support someone who may be in a bad place mentally. Predominantly it was set up so that workplaces, schools and offices can have someone who is able to identify, understand and respond to signs of mental illnesses, feelings of suicidal ideation and substance-use disorders. Most MHFA courses introduce participants to the risk factors and warning signs of mental health issues, helping them to give immediate care but also point people in the right direction for more long-term support and treatment.

I would thoroughly recommend either undertaking a course of MHFA yourself or encouraging your employer, place of work or close friends to be aware of the benefits of having someone who is trained.

3 The Zero Suicide Alliance.

This is a collaborative body of National Health Service trusts, businesses and individuals who are all committed to suicide prevention in the UK. They believe that all of us need to work together to prevent all suicides, because 'one life is one too many'.

Trying to reduce the number of suicides to zero might seem ridiculously unattainable and idealistic, but I really believe that it's a mindset and goal that we must all adopt.

On the Zero Suicide Alliance webpage, as of January 2020, there is a simple 20-minute interactive course aimed at educating members of the public in basic suicide prevention and how best to help someone who might be at risk. I would really recommend having a look at this.

4 Get political.

In the last few years, as I've said a number of times in this book, our mental health services have been cut back. Different political leaders have made pledges to change this and invest more in services, but whether or not these ever come to fruition remains to be seen. We all, however, have the chance to speak to our local MPs to demand they pressure the government into generating real and actual change.

On World Mental Health Awareness Day in October 2018, the government made Jackie Doyle-Price, MP, the UK's first ever minister for mental health and suicide prevention. I celebrated the creation of this new position with much excitement – until Jackie got to work and, to my mind, didn't make a huge impact. Sadly, she has a record of voting against LGBTQ+ rights and other human rights, which I believe often play into the many mental health issues that the most vulnerable people in society experience. So I am not entirely convinced she was the right, most compassionate and non-judgemental candidate for the job.

In July 2019 she was replaced by Nadine Dorries, MP. Now Nadine's voting record includes mostly being against LGBTQ+ rights, particularly same-sex marriage, voting for an increase in tuition fees and to scrap financial support for sixteen- to nineteen-year-olds trying to progress into further education. These two women have supposedly been our society's line of accountability for mental health and suicide failures.

I feel that a lack of equality – in terms of LGBTQ+ rights, class issues, race issues – is a big part of why there is such a broad mental health crisis in the UK. We need someone accountable for the government's policy on improving mental health services and the increasing suicide rate who also understands the full range of reasons why people are struggling today. I'd ask you to make sure you watch the work of this minister very closely and, if you don't feel like they're doing well enough, then speak out about it. You can also always write to your MP on a website called writetothem.com, to help make your voice heard about the state of our mental health services.

5 **We before me.**

Finally, I think a big thing the whole of our society can do is re-engage with a lot of community ideals and practices and to just be much kinder to one another. In the age of social media, we have become obsessed with the individual in ways that don't always generate happiness or solid foundations for relationships. There has also been a general decline in community spaces over the last few years – youth clubs have been cut, community centres shut down and many pubs have closed since the economic crash over a decade ago.

We can still create our own communities, though, and social media has been a great tool for this, but I think it's important to physically meet up with people as much as possible. Join groups, volunteer, do some fundraising for a charity – make it as fun and engaging as possible and involve any other friends or people you may know who might benefit from getting involved.

One of the best things I ever did was get involved with CALM and it's led me to so many opportunities, interesting people and like-minded friends that I wouldn't have met otherwise.

Lewis and Claire have run 10k races for CALM. Brendan has made TV shows raising awareness for their suicide prevention campaign. And Cecilia and I have continued throwing our comedy, poetry and music fundraisers to raise money for their helpline.

I feel very lucky that these guys are my best friends, so get your pals involved with any charity that's maybe helped you, and let's all try to create more action and provide more services to save the ones we love.

support

helplines, websites and more

SAMARITANS

Available 24 hours a day to provide confidential emotional support for people who are experiencing feelings of distress, despair or suicidal thoughts.

- www.samaritans.org
- 116 123 (free to call from within the UK and Ireland), 24 hours a day
- Email: jo@samaritans.org

CALM

A helpline for men and women in the UK who are down or have hit a wall for any reason, who need to talk or find information and support.

Open 5pm to midnight, every day of the year.

- www.thecalmzone.net

- Helpline for men: 0800 58 58 58
- Webchat: www.thecalmzone.net/help/webchat/

MIND

Mind offers advice, support and information to people experiencing a mental health difficulty and their family and friends. Mind also has a network of local associations in England and Wales to which people can turn for help and assistance.

Lines are open Monday to Friday, 9am to 6pm (except bank holidays).

- www.mind.org.uk
- InfoLine: 0300 123 3393 to call, or text 86463
- Email: info@mind.org.uk

PAPYRUS

PAPYRUS is the national charity dedicated to the prevention of young suicide. They support young people under thirty-five who are experiencing thoughts of suicide, as well as people concerned about someone else.

Open 10am–10pm on weekdays and 2pm–10pm on weekends and bank holidays.

- www.papyrus-uk.org
- Helpline: 0800 068 4141
- Text: 07786209697
- Email: pat@papyrus-uk.org

NHS SERVICES

Call NHS 111 (for when you need help but are not in immediate danger). Or the emergency services on 999 if you are urgently worried about someone at risk of imminent harm and in a crisis.

SHOUT TEXT LINE

Shout is the UK's first 24/7 text service, free on all major mobile networks, for anyone in crisis anytime, anywhere. It's a place to go if you're struggling to cope and you need immediate help.

Shout is powered by a team of volunteers, who are at the heart of the service.

- Text SHOUT to 85258 or visit www.giveusashout.org

THE BRITISH ASSOCIATION FOR COUNSELLING AND PSYCHOTHERAPY:

The British Association for Counselling and Psychotherapy website has a database of professional counsellors and psychotherapists practising in the UK.

- www.bacp.co.uk

SELF HARM UK

Self Harm UK are dedicated to self-harm recovery, insight and support.

- www.selfharm.co.uk

PINK THERAPY FOR LGBTQ+ PEOPLE

Pink Therapy is a directory of therapists and health professionals in the UK who identify as or are understanding of gender and sexual minorities (GSMs).

- www.pinktherapy.com

BEFRIENDERS WORLDWIDE

Befrienders Worldwide is a charity that helps people who are considering suicide or experiencing general emotional distress. They have 349 emotional support centres in over thirty countries.

- www.befrienders.org

THE ZERO SUICIDE ALLIANCE

The Zero Suicide Alliance is a collaborative of National Health Service trusts, businesses and individuals who are all committed to suicide prevention in the UK and beyond. They aim to improve support for people contemplating suicide by raising awareness of and promoting FREE suicide prevention training which is accessible to all.

The aims of this training are to: enable people to identify when someone is presenting with suicidal thoughts/ behaviour, to be able to speak out in a supportive manner, and to empower them to signpost the individual to the correct services or support. Give it a try!

- www.zerosuicidealliance.com

MENTAL HEALTH FIRST AID ENGLAND

MHFA England are an organisation to help people be trained in spotting signals of mental health issues in the workplace and beyond.

- mhfaengland.org

BLACK MINDS MATTER UK

Racial prejudice in the UK is a major contributing factor to poor mental health experienced in our communities. Black Minds Matter is a network of Black therapists who can apply their own lived experience and understanding to helping other Black people seeking help. They work and fundraise to help give black people access to therapy.

- www.blackmindsmatteruk.com

NAZ AND MATT FOUNDATION

This foundation was set up in 2014 following the sad loss of Dr Nazim Mahmood, who took his own life after his deeply religious family confronted him about his sexuality. N&M

aim to promote and protect LGBTQ+ individuals, and their friends and family by offering support and signposting them to established counselling services, to help with challenges linked to sexuality or gender identity where religion may be affecting the situation.

- www.nazandmattfoundation.org

CRUSE BEREAVEMENT CARE

Cruse Bereavement Care is the leading national charity for bereaved people. They help both those affected by grief as well as employers, friends and family wanting to support someone.

They also tailor specific services and resources to helping those affected by specific tragedies, such as acts of terrorism, public accidents, or resources on how to grieve in isolation due to the COVID-19 pandemic.

- www.cruse.org.uk/get-help
- Free Helpline: 0808 808 1677

Acknowledgements

Firstly, thank you, Mum, for making me laugh and cooking me roasts anytime this book got too much for me.

Thank you my super-star agents, Gordon Wise and Kat Buckle at Curtis Brown, for helping this book even be a thing. You have both kept me sane, taken me for posh lunches, Pret lunches, and talked through everything with me whenever my anxiety flared up badly. I can't thank you both enough.

A HUGE thank you to Yvonne Jacob at Penguin for wanting this book and giving it so much love and time and attention. You are brilliant!

To Nell Warner for being so patient and kind as I hacked away.

And to the genius of Liz Marvin – whose notes made me laugh, cry, spiral into panic, ascend into joy and feel all the breadth of human emotions one can possibly feel about a memoir. Thank you so much.

Whilst I was writing I had two pieces of sad news about family members that made it quite tough to write this book at times, and Yvonne and everyone at Penguin were completely amazing in supporting me. I cannot thank them enough for putting their money where their mouth is when it comes to genuinely caring about the mental wellbeing of their writers. Thank you also to Siofra and Alice for having faith in this project and comforting me in meetings, when I'd be like 'WHAT AM I DOING WRITING A BOOK!?!??'

To the charity CALM – I cannot thank you enough for what you've done for me in the past decade. Staff members past and present, including Rachel Clare, Paul Shiels, Jane Powell and Rachel Stephenson, among many other names, all of whom have supported me over the years I've worked with CALM and who have made that charity grow into a nationally recognised campaign. Thank you, crew, you're incredible!

To my pal Nicola Coughlan, who is actually the reason this book even exists in your hands. Thank you for making sure Yvonne at Penguin came to see my Edinburgh show in 2017 and thank you for putting up with my frantic WhatsApp messages whilst I was writing this book. You're my fave 'wee lesbian'.

To my pals, Lewis, Cecilia, Lucy, Inez, Izzy, Brendan, Dave, Claire, Ben, Dom, Steven, Maria, Owen, Patrick, Lolly, Cam, Alex, Jack, Ruth, Georgia, Camille, Holly, Laura, Gabe, Adelaide and Brendan, Jon, Sarah (you all sound like an awful Year 2 class when I type your names together) and anyone I've forgotten (I'm so tired, I've just written a book!). All of them have had me panic ring them over the past eighteen months or have heard me wanging on and on about working on this project and all have continually told me to cheer the fuck up and carry the fuck on. THANK YOU!!

To Bob Boyton, for letting me take up swathes of kitchen table space with books and notes and for always giving me a supportive wave 'goodnight' when I'd still be up late typing. Thank you for everything you've done for me.

To Scarlett Curtis, for having me in the *It's Not OK to Be Blue* book and for having faith in my writing and what I have to say about a sometimes very frustrating mental health world. You are utterly brilliant.

To the Roundhouse and Soho Theatre for always being incredibly supportive of my writing from as far back as my teens. I would encourage any young writers or comedians to look at the amazing work both Roundhouse and Soho do with young people across London and the UK.

Thanks also to Underbelly and Sarah Sanders at Arts Council England for helping give me my big break at the Edinburgh festival and essentially putting me on a path to a career in writing and performing. Likewise, thank you to BBC Comedy, Radio 4 and BBC Three for being the first to give that work a big platform.

Thank you to Patrick Stoddart and Jim McClellan at Westminster University's journalism department for supporting me, even beyond my graduation. You two are legends and without that course and scholarship I would never have met Olly and never figured out so much about myself.

And, finally, to Olly, my dad and my nan, Sicely. Thinking of you every day. Thanks for all the wise words. Hope this makes you proud xxx